HYPNOBIRTH

Evidence, practice and support for birth professionals

Teri Gavin-Jones and Sandra Handford

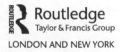

Routledge
Taylor & Francis Group

LONDON AND NEW YORK

First published 2016
by Routledge
2 Park Square, Milton Park, Abingdon, Oxon OX14 4RN

and by Routledge
711 Third Avenue, New York, NY 10017

Routledge is an imprint of the Taylor & Francis Group, an informa business

British Library Cataloguing in Publication Data
A catalogue record for this book is available from the British Library

Library of Congress Cataloging in Publication Data
Names: Gavin-Jones, Teri, author. | Handford, Sandra, author.
Title: Hypnobirth : evidence, practice and support for birth professionals / Teri Gavin-Jones and Sandra Handford.
Description: Abingdon, Oxon ; New York, NY : Routledge, 2016. | Includes bibliographical references and index.
Identifiers: LCCN 2015040933| ISBN 9781138900561 (hbk) | ISBN 9781138900578 (pbk.) | ISBN 9781315707174 (ebk)
Subjects: | MESH: Hypnosis. | Labor Pain--therapy. | Parturition. | Pregnancy. | Prenatal Education.
Classification: LCC RG526 | NLM WQ 300 | DDC 618.2--dc23
LC record available at http://lccn.loc.gov/2015040933

ISBN: 978-1-138-90056-1 (hbk)
ISBN: 978-1-138-90057-8 (pbk)
ISBN: 978-1-315-70717-4 (ebk)

Typeset in Bembo
by Taylor & Francis Books

Printed and bound by CPI Group (UK) Ltd, Croydon, CR0 4YY

HYPNOBIRTH

Maternity services and choices for labour and birth are fast evolving. Hypnobirth involves preparation for childbirth using tried and tested hypnotherapy techniques in harmony with midwifery best practices, and increasing numbers of women are turning to the technique.

Written by two experienced practitioners, this is the first evidence-based practice book for health professionals on this subject. Chapters include coverage of:

- what hypnosis is and the history of hypnobirth;
- the power of the mind and the effect of language;
- relaxation and breathing techniques;
- the neocortex and hormones;
- birth partners, relationships, women's advocates and primary supporters.

Throughout the book, the authors provide professionals working in clinical midwifery practice with information and evidence-based findings to support the use of hypnobirth. The book includes case studies, scripts and reflective questions to encourage a deeper understanding of the techniques and issues and to engage and inspire the reader.

Hypnobirth is essential reading for midwives, obstetricians, student midwives, doulas and any practitioner involved in preparing and supporting pregnant women for labour.

Teri Gavin-Jones is a specialist midwife in parent education for Colchester Hospital University Foundation Trust. Teri trained with and taught for the National Childbirth Trust as an antenatal teacher for ten years. She is an active birth teacher and water birth specialist. She undertakes monthly midwifery training on normal birth and is a guest lecturer at Anglia Ruskin University, UK, in parent education. She is a hypnobirth trainer and co-founder of Hypnobirth Midwives UK which delivers in-house hypnobirth training for midwives at hospital trusts across the UK. Teri has spoken at conferences both in the UK and abroad on hypnobirth and the future of parent education in the NHS.

Sandra Handford is a member of the British Institute of Hypnotherapy and Psychotherapy and is registered with the Complementary and Natural Healthcare Council (CNHC). She is a co-founder of Hypnobirth Midwives UK and teaches Hypnosis for Hypnobirthing in-house to midwives in hospital trusts across the country.

Transforming birth together

CONTENTS

ILLUSTRATIONS

Figures

Tables

Boxes

FOREWORD

There is no doubt in many birth practitioners' minds (and that includes midwives, doulas, childbirth educators and obstetricians) that childbirth in high-income countries is approaching a tipping point – either towards an escalating trend to higher and higher caesarean section rates or a profound rediscovery of the power and wonder of birth physiology. Recent guidance on place of birth in the United Kingdom recommending for the first time in many generations a turn back to homely, low-tech places and spaces like midwifery units and home has certainly caught the headlines. For natural birth enthusiasts this is 'manna from heaven' but many are asking, can midwives and birth companions support this shift in the numbers anticipated (possibly between 30 and 40 per cent of all births) when they have been trained and practised in the industrial birthing model of large maternity units? Will women embrace these options when they are exposed to a diet of frightening, emergency-esque reality TV childbirth?

So there could not be a more opportune time for two experienced practitioners of hypnobirth to introduce women, childbirth attendants and the wider public to an accessible, common-sense, informative guide to hypnosis in childbirth.

Their book, written in plain English, is full of all the background information to enable those new to hypnobirth to understand this emerging therapy/approach/ science that is making a significant impact on the childbirth landscape. What's great about their style is the absence of an 'in-your face' evangelical fervour and rather extravagant claims that characterise other books. They are convincing about the case for hypnobirthing but this is based on a considered, beautifully built argument from history, childbirth anthropology, neuro-endocrine-psycho-physiological evidence and an emerging evidence base from direct research studies. They also discuss the topic against the backdrop of the central premise of relational-based care, so fundamental for a positive childbirth experience.

Towards the end of the book, the authors explore the vexed question of labour pain in an illuminating, realistic and pragmatic way.

This is not a textbook of hypnobirth but a lucid, stimulating and timely introduction and I highly recommend it. It will reward the reader with insight, information and practical advice, and is especially relevant for childbearing women and childbirth professionals.

Dr Denis Walsh
Associate Professor in Midwifery
Nottingham University, UK

PREFACE

In 2011 we embarked on a mission to introduce hypnobirth into a National Health Service (NHS) Trust. We were only the second hospital to do this in the UK. We had been encountering women using hypnobirth techniques in labour and, although the benefits were obvious, it's fair to say that there was some suspicion and anxiety surrounding hypnobirth. As we introduced the course programme, we modified it to included labour physiology, active birth, rebozo and massage, along with recognised hypnosis techniques. The uptake was slow and steady, but the results impressive. Women and their birth partners became almost evangelical about the experience. Even when birth did not go to plan, hypnobirth enabled them to remain calm, focused and positive.

The year 2015 saw our Trust with 26 trained hypnobirthing midwives, the most in the country to date. We began to realise the impact that hypnobirth had on the women's experience, their birth outcomes and their antenatal journey. It has been offered free to all women since the beginning of 2015, and currently an average of 25 per cent of our pregnant population use hypnosis for labour. Hypnobirth has replaced standard antenatal classes as the demand has grown in popularity. NHS Trusts across the UK are realising the benefit, and we frequently train other NHS Trusts with an in-house programme. Their results are just as impressive.

As the popularity of hypnobirth in the UK continues to grow, the question over its effectiveness remains. Women report varying results, some experiencing a pain-free easy birth, whilst others feel it to be ineffective. Hypnobirth courses do vary, and we believe there needs to be a balance of good quality antenatal education coupled with tried and tested hypnosis techniques. Some women access private practitioners who are not medically trained. Some access it through hypnotherapy. Others buy a book and CD and call it hypnobirthing. This variation may result in difficulty assessing the effectiveness.

The use of hypnosis for childbirth is not new. Grantly Dick-Read was writing about this subject in the 1930s, and his popular book, *Childbirth without Fear* (2004), introduced the fear–tension–pain cycle. Many midwives remember teaching antenatal classes and teaching 'the breathing'. Being involved with the National Childbirth Trust (NCT) as a teacher in the 1990s, it was all about the breathing. However, moving into the NHS as a midwife a few years later there was a noticeable absence of breathing being taught. One midwife, when questioned about learning breathing techniques by a pregnant woman, responded with 'well you won't stop breathing in labour!' There seemed to be a divide between women who needed to learn some skills, and midwives who put little faith in self-help techniques. Breathing was very much out of fashion.

Hypnobirth has brought 'the breathing' back into popular culture. What goes around comes around, and nothing is truly original. What is unique is the package that hypnobirth offers to women and birth partners. Hypnobirth offers much more than breathing techniques and is a complete antenatal course. As a midwife, childbirth educator, doula or hypnobirth practitioner, you may feel that NHS antenatal education falls a little short. In most instances you would be right. Hypnobirth is the course that redresses the balance. We have seen the rewards of couples working together, understanding birth physiology and experiencing some truly remarkable births. This book aims to explain the principles, deepen your understanding of hypnosis and enable you to support women and birth partners through a hypnobirthing labour. We believe hypnobirth is the future for antenatal education. Once you have witnessed it, we think you will too.

2015

Reference

Dick-Read, G. (2004). *Childbirth without fear. The principles and practices of natural childbirth.* London, Pinter and Martin (first published by Heinemann Medical Books in 1942).

1

THE HISTORY OF ANTENATAL EDUCATION

From Mothercraft to the National Childbirth Trust (NCT)

In 1918, Dr Truby King established 'mothercraft' training, focusing on the value of pre-parenting and breastfeeding. The Mothercraft Training Society was the fore-runner of antenatal education in the UK. King George V knighted Dr King as mothercraft education spread and, in 1927, the *British Journal of Nursing* wrote about the Mothercraft movement:

'It is [sic] the duty of every mother to fit herself for the perfect fulfilment of the natural calls of motherhood, both before and after childbirth, and especially to advocate and promote the breastfeeding of infants.'

The duty of women in 1927 was to raise children within marriage and the law of the church. Education for women around the subject of childbirth was unheard of at this time.

The *British Journal of Nursing* states: 'to teach them to fear God, and to honour the King, to be loyal citizens, and to share in the duties and responsibilities of the community. What higher destiny can a woman desire?' (RCN Archive, 1927).

The introduction of the National Health Service (NHS) in 1948 enabled maternity services to be offered to all women. Pre-war health insurance schemes had left women and children particularly vulnerable. Maternal mortality rates had risen in England and Wales between 1900 and 1937 to over 40 deaths per 10,000 births. After 1948 this rate steadily declined (Davis, 2013).

The idea of a more natural birthing experience was pioneered by English obstetrician Dr Grantly Dick-Read. He had experienced a conversation with a woman living in Whitechapel in the 1920s that childbirth was not meant to be painful, leading the young Dick-Read to dedicate his life to exploring natural childbirth. Dick-Read was early to suggest the 'fear–tension–pain' cycle in his work, *Natural Childbirth* (1933). He argued that, when we are afraid during childbirth, the body draws blood away from non-vital organs, such as the uterus, to the extremities, which results in pain. By removing fear and its physiological consequence, the uterus can function as intended, eliminating extreme pain. Breaking or removing this pain cycle is a central concept in hypnobirth.

In contrast to Dick-Read's exploration of childbirth, the NHS began offering mothercraft classes to women in the 1950s. This would involve advice on pregnancy (no swimming, but cigarettes were fine) and practical advice on baby care. There was no information about the actual birth and certainly no advice on coping with labour.

Inspired by the writings of Dick-Read, the Natural Childbirth Association (NCA) was founded in 1956 by Prunella Briance. She placed an advert in the personal columns of the *The Daily Telegraph*, and *The Times*, inviting interest in the formation of an association to promote and better understand the Dick-Read system of natural childbirth. She received overwhelming interest and support. There were early years of conflict between the medical profession and the NCA, but eventually in 1961 it obtained charitable status and became the National Childbirth Trust (NCT).

Lamaze and the Bradley Method

Whilst the NCT was being formed in the UK, in France, in 1951, Dr Fernand Lamaze was introducing childbirth education that he had originally observed in

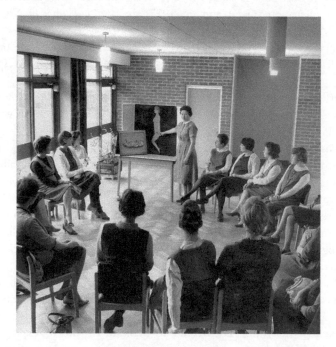

FIGURE 1.1 1960s midwife with mothers-to-be
Source: Photo courtesy of the QNI; copyright Barnet Saidman

Russia. The Soviet Union was routinely using psychoprophylaxis as an alternative to analgesia for pain relief. Here, women were not choosing the method, but were forced to use it by a central government that was unwilling to provide access to obstetric analgesia. Lamaze had travelled to the Soviet Union after hearing Soviet obstetrician Anatoly Petrovich Nikolaev speak at an international congress. Lamaze was given permission to observe birth in Soviet Russia and went on to say that he wept with joy at witnessing a woman giving birth with no sign of pain or discomfort. Lamaze returned to Paris and sought to implement psychoprophylaxis techniques. He joined forces with obstetrician Pierre Vellay and kinesiologist André Bourrel to establish the first obstetric prophylactic clinic in the West in 1952.

By the early 1960s France and the United States were discovering psychoprophylaxis. In an effort to distance it from Russia, the method was named the Lamaze method. Elizabeth Bing was a childbirth educator teaching the Dick-Read method in New York. Bing contacted Marjorie Karmel, who had given birth assisted by Dr Lamaze. Karmel was an American woman in Paris who had sought the help of Lamaze to birth her first child. She was so enamoured with the experience that she wrote a book – *Thank you, Dr Lamaze* (1959). Together Bing and Karmel founded the American Society for Psychoprophylaxis in Obstetrics in 1960, later becoming Lamaze International. Michaels (2014) describes the typical woman drawn to this method as 'well-educated, married, white, middle and upper-class'. Some might say that until very recently the NCT has also attracted this demographic in the UK.

Alongside the popularity of the Lamaze method, the Bradley Method was being conceived. Robert A. Bradley, a Denver obstetrician, developed 'husband-coached childbirth' in 1947, publishing his first book in 1965 (Bradley, 2008). The method claims that, of over 1,000,000 couples trained in The Bradley Method, over 86 per cent of them have had spontaneous, unmedicated vaginal births. Bradley was a pioneer in including men in the childbirth process and expanding the husband's role into birth coaching. Childbirth preparation across the continents was evolving and adapting to women's needs. However, the combination of breathing techniques, relaxation and childbirth education has much in common with hypnobirth today.

As women in the UK continued to seek education and choice, the role of the National Childbirth Trust as a provider of information became pronounced. By the 1970s childbirth was more medicalised than ever. The Peel Report (Department of Health and Social Security, 1970) resulted in almost all birth taking place in a hospital setting. The NCT was a vocal critic of routine medicalisation and became increasingly polarised from some of the medical profession. The allegiance between many midwives, pregnant couples and the NCT was building in strength. The NCT published its first research into mothers' experience of induction of labour, and women were looking toward it as a source of information as well as support.

Women's rights for birth – 1960s to the 1980s

The 1960s to the 1980s were times of great change and a growing awareness of women's rights for birth. Authors such as Sally Inch, Marjorie Tew and Sheila

Kitzinger added to the weight of evidence for women-centred care. Frederick Leboyer's *Birth without Violence* (1974) began to focus the attention on the birth room environment and considered birth from the baby's perspective. French obstetrician Michel Odent added to the concept of natural birthing, introducing birthing pools and exploring the impact of the birth environment. Janet Balaskas and Yehudi Gordon pioneered the active birth movement, which is still as relevant today. The Society for the Prevention of Cruelty to Pregnant Women, founded in 1960, quickly renamed itself the Association for Improvements in the Maternity Services (AIMS), and The Association of Radical Midwives (ARM) was formed. It says much about maternity services today that these organisations are as well used and necessary as they were then.

Beverley Beech writing for AIMS in 2011 comments,

> letters women wrote in the 1960s are little different from letters written today. Maternity care is dominated by obstetricians who have moved from a position where they were called in to assist with a problem labour to the current situation where they control the majority of pregnancies and births.

As far as the evolution of women's choice since the 1960s, there is clearly much work still to be done. This also applies to antenatal education. Classes on offer today are limited to NHS or private sector classes. Research suggests that many NHS classes are of poor quality and do not provide the small interactive sessions that couples are looking for (Barlow et al., 2009). A review of maternity services conducted by the Commission for Healthcare Audit and Inspection (2008) found that antenatal education was not being adequately addressed by many trusts. It found that 86 per cent of trusts offered first-time mothers an opportunity to attend classes; 71 per cent of trusts offered classes to mothers who had previously given birth; 15 per cent of women reported the classes were not at a convenient time of day; 28 per cent of women reported that there were an insufficient number of classes in the course; and 20 per cent of women reported that the classes did not cover the topics that women wanted.

The expectations of pregnant women and their families is that within the pregnancy there will be some kind of antenatal education. This may be within an NHS setting and taught by midwives (sometimes referred to as 'parentcraft') or women may seek private sector classes.

Whilst research into antenatal education remains limited in comparison to other areas of childbirth, what is known is that good birth preparation is of value. Research published in 2009 stated: 'Participation in antenatal preparation courses can be associated with higher satisfaction with the birth experience.'

'When birth partners are well prepared for their role, a woman's experience of birth is likely to be more positive' (Schrader McMillan and Stuart-Brown, 2009).

Although the research into this area of pregnancy is comparatively new, the findings have not reached a wider audience. Many women and their partners do not understand or appreciate the benefit of attending antenatal classes. Male birth partners fear that the classes will be uncomfortable, irrelevant to them and women focused. It may be that, given the poor quality of the traditional NHS antenatal class, both midwives and parents feel that they are of little value.

Antenatal education today

The Department of Health published a document in 2011, 'Preparation for birth and beyond'. This document is unique in addressing the relationship between pregnancy and its impact on later health outcomes. 'From pregnancy onwards, the relationship between a baby and his or her primary caregiver has a lasting impact on that child's future, including on his or her health as an adult.'

The same document also discusses the difficulty of the NHS providing antenatal classes, describing a 'narrow focus' on the process of giving birth. This has historically been the divide between NHS and NCT classes. The NCT has offered a product where small groups of participants explore birth in an unhurried, friendly atmosphere. Couples value the time to discuss issues and the lasting friendships often made. NHS 'parentcraft' classes are seen as second rate. The name 'parentcraft' is a modification on 'mothercraft' when it became apparent that fathers would like to be included. The fact that the NHS still uses the 1960s name to describe an antenatal class says a lot about progress and evolution. Antenatal education is unreported in national statistics, with some hospitals offering a lot, and some offering nothing. In certain parts of the UK, classes have been cut or the service withdrawn as a result of financial restraints (Clift-Matthews, 2007).

Redshaw and Heikkila (2010) showed that in England most NHS antenatal classes were offered in the North-East (73 per cent) and fewest classes were offered in the East Midlands (62 per cent). Tomintz et al. (2013) state that, although the NHS provides classes free of charge, a shortage of staff and resources means a limited universal provision of such services.

Providing antenatal classes within the NHS is problematic and multifaceted. Constraints such as funding, adequate training and resource allocation all have an impact on the provision of classes. From an organisational perspective, antenatal classes historically have been seen as non-essential work and therefore are undervalued. Midwives themselves are reluctant to teach classes and can feel unprepared. Midwifery education to teach classes is minimal, and student midwives receive their learning from other community midwives teaching classes. What the community midwife delivers in a class is often up to her. Few hospital trusts have parent education leads, and often there is no standardised teaching plan. This results in information of varying quality. Is it right that a midwifery qualification automatically translates into a teaching qualification? Most community midwives working in a team are just relieved that someone else is doing it and the box for parent education is ticked.

One online blogger writes:

> NHS classes: free but a total waste of time. Around 40 individuals and couples in a theatre-style auditorium. During question and answer sessions she couldn't

really hear what other participants were saying and they ran out of handouts. Pain relief methods were discussed briefly as more or less a list of options.

(Smurthwaite, 2009)

Often time constraints within the hospital classes result in a narrow topic – the pain relief menu. Women and their partners arrive at classes expecting to learn pain management techniques. These may not necessarily be focused on analgesia, but self-help techniques such as massage, breathing, active birth, waterbirth and rebozo. These take time to teach and time to learn, and NHS classes are short on time and resources. The NHS class facilitator dictates the class content. If she/he is not confident in teaching holistic pain management techniques, they will be sidelined. The question is raised, do health professionals see value in teaching skills such as breathing techniques, massage and active birth? Is value only seen in pharmacology?

The introduction of hypnosis in childbirth

It is within this landscape that hypnobirth has emerged as an antenatal course to meet the needs of couples. Although initially a private, paid-for course, many healthcare trusts are seeing the value of replacing the outdated parentcraft with hypnobirth.

There has been some discussion as to who actually coined the term hypno-birthing. Two American women both began to use it in the 1980s and have been instrumental in the spread of hypnobirthing: Michelle Leclaire O'Neill, whose work was partly based on Dick-Read's research and Marie Mongan, who founded The HypnoBirthing Institute in America.

Whilst the American Mongan method began to filter slowly into the UK in the '80s, it has gained momentum and pace in the last 5 years. Within the UK, British versions of hypnobirth were founded. Natal Hypnotherapy, KG Hypnobirthing, HypnobirthMidwivesUK and Wise Hippo have all contributed to the growing industry.

As a team midwife, hypnobirth came to my attention in 2008. A small amount of women were birthing in the hospital using the techniques. There were mut-terings from the midwives of not being able to use the word pain, birthing in the dark and not being able to talk to the woman. The general feeling was that it was odd and probably would not work. The handover room can be a wealth of poli-tically incorrect labels: the NCT woman, the one with the birth plan, the teacher, the VBAC (vaginal birth after caesarean), and now we had the hypnobirther!

Hypnobirth in the NHS

The percentage of women using hypnobirth was small, but the increase was steady. By 2011 the interest had grown and we decided to bring hypnobirth 'in house'. The women using the techniques had all been taught by private practitioners, and we saw the value of having hypnobirth combined with midwifery information. We trained three midwives and began offering hypnobirth as a paid-for course in the summer of 2011.

Analgesia for Vaginal Births 2011

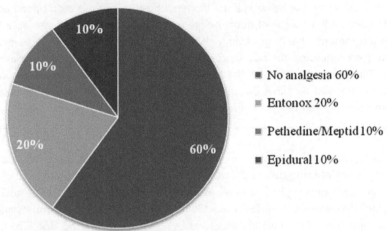

FIGURE 1.2 Audit 2011: 30 women − 27 primigravid women; 3 multigravid women
Source: Gavin-Jones, T., 2011: Colchester Hospital Hypnobirth audit

In the first year of hypnobirth the numbers were small. We offered one course a month, but this was not always full. The first audit of hypnobirth was August 2011 until April 2012. (See Fig. 1.2.) There were 30 women in total: 27 women were first-time mums; 3 were second-time. The vaginal birth rate was 90 per cent; 14 per cent were assisted birth. The 10 per cent caesarean section rate was 2 in-labour caesarean birth and 1 planned breech caesarean birth. The interesting figures are the use of analgesia and the length of labour. A total of 59 per cent of women used no pharmacological drugs at all. And 55 per cent of women gave birth in less than 6 hours. More important was the feedback, not only from the women but from the birth partners. There were stories of working as a partnership, being fully involved and, most importantly, of birth satisfaction, whatever the outcome.

BOX 1.1 LISA AND JODY'S STORY

The hypnobirth teaching was professional and informal and never patronising. We learnt lots of new skills together as a couple, which I think actually helped us to bond and grow closer too, as Jody felt so much more a part of our pregnancy. Some of the techniques we will use in other areas of our lives (dealing with stress, insomnia, etc.).

I think the hypnobirth techniques made a huge difference to our birth experience, mostly because I felt confident about what was going on inside my body (so didn't feel panicky) and also because Jody had been given lots of tools to help keep us both calm and focused.

When we were admitted to the birthing suite, Jody spent some time setting up the room with aromatherapy oils, coloured LED candles, dimming the lights, laying out blankets and treats and putting my playlist on the sound dock. It felt more like being in a spa than in a hospital room. I didn't need any pain relief until a couple of hours before our baby was born, as I was able to breathe through the surges calmly. When I started getting the urge to bear down, we requested the birthing pool, which felt amazing and really relaxed me. The whole way through the birth our baby's heartbeat remained strong and healthy and he came out quite happily in the pool, just under 10 hours from when we had first been admitted.

By 2014 the number of women requesting hypnobirth had increased dramatically. We were offering three courses a month alongside standard antenatal classes. Often demand outweighed supply. Another snapshot audit in 2014 used 78 hypnobirthing women. (See Fig. 1.3.) Of these, 67 were first-time mums and 11 were second-time. No analgesia was used by 27 per cent of the first births, and 28 per cent of subsequent births used no analgesia.

Dartford and Gravesham NHS Trust introduced hypnobirth in 2014. During March 2014–February 2015, 191 women attended the hypnobirth course. Of these, 79 per cent were first births. They evaluated the impact of hypnosis on pain management and found 36 per cent of women used hypnobirth strategies alone. A total of 95 per cent of women experienced a first stage of less than 6 hours. The remaining 5 per cent were averaging a first stage of 6.94 hours.

As more NHS hospitals become involved in offering hypnobirth as part of their parent education programme, statistics can be collected and compared. There does seem to be a trend for shorter labours and less use of analgesia. This will have an effect on the woman's recovery, her length of stay and how she feels about the experience.

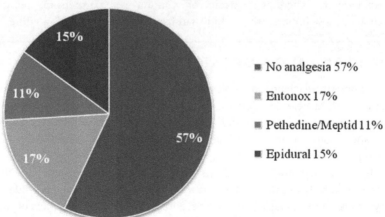

Analgesia for Vaginal Births 2014

- No analgesia 57%
- Entonox 17%
- Pethedine/Meptid 11%
- Epidural 15%

FIGURE 1.3 Audit 2014: 78 women – 67 primigravid women; 11 multigravid women
Source: Gavin-Jones, T., 2014: Colchester Hospital Hypnobirth audit

Many antenatal programmes come and go. A quick internet search will reveal a multitude of private practitioners offering pregnancy yoga and Pilates, and many midwives, NCT teachers and doulas offering antenatal classes. Hypnobirth seems to have caught the imagination of the pregnant population and has grown in popularity at speed.

What is important is that hypnobirth techniques, whatever the programme, deliver the same results. The scripts will vary. The 'brand' will vary, but the hypnosis will work. For many couples, the NHS branding is recognised and respected, and a hypnobirth course within the NHS offers a powerful tool for change.

References

Barlow, J., Coe, C., Redshaw, M. and Underdown, A. (2009). *Birth and beyond: Stakeholder perceptions of current antenatal education provision in England*. London: Department of Health. Available at: http://webarchive.nationalarchives.gov.uk/20130107105354/http://www.dh. gov.uk/prod_consum_dh/groups/dh_digitalassets/documents/digitalasset/dh_109831.pdf.

Beech, B. (2011). Challenging the medicalisation of birth. *AIMS*, October 2nd: aims.org.uk/ Journal/Vol23No2/challengingmedicalisation. Retrieved July 22nd 2015.

Bradley, Robert A. (2008). *Husband coached childbirth*. New York: Bantam Books (first published in 1965 by Harper and Row).

Clift-Matthews, V. (2007). Maternity services suffer again. *British Journal of Midwifery*, 184.

Commission for Healthcare Audit and Inspection (2008). *Towards a better birth: A review of maternity services in England*. London: Commission for Healthcare Audit and Inspection.

Davis, A. (2013). Choice, policy and practice in maternity care since 1948. *History and Policy*, May 30: www.historyandpolicy.org/policy-papers/papers/choice-policy-and-practice-in-maternity-care-since-1948. Retrieved January 31st 2015.

Department of Health (2011). *Preparation for birth and beyond: A resource pack for leaders of community groups and activities*. Available at: https://www.gov.uk/government/publications/preparation-for-birth-and-beyond-a-resource-pack-for-leaders-of-community-groups-and-activities.

Department of Health and Social Security (1970). *Domiciliary midwifery and maternity bed needs: The report of the Standing Maternity and Midwifery Advisory Committee (Sub-committee Chairman J. Peel)*. London: HMSO.

Dick-Read, G. (1933). *Natural childbirth*. London: Heinemann Medical Books.

Karmel, M. (1959). *Thank you, Dr Lamaze*. London: Pinter and Martin.

Leboyer, F. (1974). *Birth without violence*. Glasgow: William Collins and Son.

Michaels, P. A. (2014). *Lamaze. An international history*. Oxford: Oxford University Press.

Redshaw, M. and Heikkila, K. (2010). *Delivered with care: A national survey of women's experience of maternity care*. Oxford: National Perinatal Epidemiology Unit, University of Oxford.

Royal College of Nursing Archive (1927). rcn.org.uk, April: http://rcnarchive.rcn.org.uk/data/ VOLUME075-1927/page086-volume75-april1927.pdf. Retrieved July 9th 2014.

Schrader McMillan, A. and Stuart-Brown, S. (2009). *Home and community based parenting support programs and interventions*. Warwick: Warwick University. Available at: http://wrap.warwick. ac.uk/3239/1/WRAP_Stewart_brown_DataPrev_final_12_03_10_AS__(2)_(2).pdf.

Smurthwaite, K. (2009). *The truth about antenatal classes*. The F Word blog, May 27: www. thefword.org.uk/2009/05/truth_about_antenatal. Retrieved August 19th 2015.

Tomintz, M., Clarke, G., Rigby, J. and Green, J. (2013). Optimising the location of antenatal classes. *Midwifery*, 33–43.

2

WHAT IS HYPNOSIS?

A brief history of hypnosis

Hypnosis, in one form or another, can be traced back over 4,000 years to the sleep temples of Imhotep in ancient Egypt and later in ancient Greece (Ellenberger, 1981). Imhotep, who lived in the twenty-seventh century BC, was vizier, architect, priest and physician to the Third Dynasty Pharaoh Djoser and was responsible for the Step Pyramid at Saqqara. Imhotep is the first known physician who did not include magic in his healing practice. In 1892, Sir William Osler described Imhotep as 'the first figure of a physician to stand out clearly from the mists of antiquity' (Osler, 1892). After his death, Imhotep was given divine status by the Egyptian people (Colgan, 2012). The Ancient Greeks identified Imhotep with Asklepios, their god of healing. Asklepios was the son of Apollo and a prominent mortal called Coronis. According to mythology, Coronis died giving birth to Asklepios, and Apollo cut the baby out of the womb. Apollo entrusted Asklepios to the care of Chiron, a centaur, who educated people in the art of medicine, including Hippocrates, Achilles and Hercules.

Asklepios became renowned for healing, bringing people back from the brink of death, and even resurrection. His miraculous healings led him to be considered a demi-god for whom people built extravagant temples, the eldest of which was the Temple of Asklepios at Epidauros, built in the fifth century BC.

People would embark on pilgrimages to one of the temples, which were often in major city states, taking a clay votive of their ailing body part as a symbol of their sickness, which they gave to the priest. At Pergamum, an inscription shows that, following a purification procedure, elaborate rituals and fasting were used to bring patients into a trance state before being questioned by the priests. 'After three more days without food, the patient would be susceptible to suggestion' (Cilliers and Retief, 2013). This can be seen as an early use of suggestion and hypnosis in health.

The patient would then spend the night in the abaton, the holiest room in the temple, to sleep and hopefully dream. The dreams were likely to have been influenced by all that they had seen in the temple and the rituals they had undertaken. The following day the priest would interpret these dreams and suggest a remedy or would prescribe a course of action.

Animal magnetism and the mesmerists

Hypnosis, as we know it today, is generally considered to come from the theory of animal magnetism, or mesmerism, popular in the eighteenth century. Franz Anton Mesmer (1734–1815) was born in Germany and studied philosophy, theology and law in Vienna, before studying medicine. He believed that an invisible fluid connected everything in the universe and that the planets in the solar system had a magnetic effect on all living things. Mesmer called this invisible fluid animal magnetism.

In their book *Animal Magnetism*, Alfred Binet and Charles Féré (1888), describe how, during the Middle Ages, magnets had been observed to possess healing properties. They recount how the 'first trace of this belief appears in the works of Paracelsus' the early-fourteenth-century physician, alchemist and astrologer. Binet and Féré report how Mesmer took this principle and applied it to 'the sick by means of contact and of passes'.

Mesmer believed that, when this magnetic field was out of balance, it caused illness and disease in the human body and that the application of magnets would restore balance and provide a cure. As his work developed, he theorised that, as this invisible fluid connected everything, it was unnecessary to apply magnets directly to the body, but that certain people had the ability to control this invisible fluid. Mesmer also hypothesised that a patient holding a bottle of magnetised water could be cured and that magnets themselves were not necessary. Mesmer would sometimes touch his patients with a magnetic wand or make sweeping gestures to direct the flow of the magnetic fluid; these were known as 'passes'. Mesmer also discovered that there must be a close connection or harmony between physician and patient, or *rapport*, as it is known in French.

In 1777, Mesmer treated a young woman called Maria Theresa Paradis, who had become blind as a young child. Her parents introduced her to music to enrich her life, and she became an accomplished musician and singer. After seeing her perform at the age of 11, the Queen-Empress Maria Theresa, wife of Holy Roman Emperor Francis I, became her patron. The Empress provided her with a pension so that she could continue her musical education. Although, under Mesmer's treatment, Miss Paradis recovered some sight, she became very agitated and lost her confidence to perform. A few months after her parents had stopped the treatments, her family reported that she was blind once more and prone to convulsions. Mesmer claimed that her parents had had a conflict of interest and had forced her to imitate both the convulsions and the blindness, in order to retain her pension. As a result, Mesmer's popularity waned and he decided to leave Vienna.

In 1778, Mesmer moved to Paris. He was a very charismatic and theatrical man who wore a silk, lilac coat and used a magnetic wand. He became a favourite amongst the aristocracy and quickly built a large, lucrative practice. Mesmer would often hold group healing sessions. Binet and Féré describe how several rows of patients would sit or stand around a 'baquet' all holding hands and joined together by a rope. The baquet was a large oak vat, filled with magnetised water, with bent metal rods protruding through the wooden top. Patients would press the diseased part of their body against these metal rods. The lighting would be dim and soft, and ethereal music would play. Whilst walking around the group, Mesmer would speak in low tones, sometimes touching an individual with his wand, although he preferred to use his hands to direct the magnetic flow when working with young women. The participants would listen and become entranced by the experience and some would convulse and claim a miraculous cure. Convulsive crises became synonymous with mesmerism. Mesmer used his powers of relaxation and sugges- tion so successfully that we still use the words *mesmerised* and *mesmerism* today to describe this effect.

Mesmer trained others who used animal magnetism and it became widely practised in parts of Britain and Europe, with some practitioners travelling as far as America.

The Franklin Commission

Although Mesmer had many followers, he also had his detractors especially among orthodox physicians whose patients were drawn to Mesmer. In 1784, King Louis XVI requested that the government investigate the legitimacy of Mesmer's claims. Two Royal Commissions of Inquiry were set up to evaluate the practice of animal magnetism; the more prestigious group included such important names as:

- Benjamin Franklin – diplomat, scientist and America's Minister Plenipotentiary to France
- Jean-Sylvain Bailly – astronomer
- Michel Joseph Majault – physician
- Jean d'Arcet – physician and chemist
- Gabriel de Bory – geographer and cartographer
- Joseph-Ignace Guillotin – physician
- Antoine-Laurent Lavoisier – chemist.

The Franklin Commission was able to successfully recreate the effects attributed to animal magnetism simply by the manipulation of the subject's imagination, but discovered that magnetism alone would not recreate these effects without the imagination. The Commission concluded that the effects attributed to animal magnetism were due to the subject's expectations and imagination. The commis- sioners also acknowledged that imagination and suggestion might be used in a positive, therapeutic manner (Lanska and Lanska, 2007). Dr Benjamin Rush, eminent physician and friend of Benjamin Franklin, rejected Mesmer's explanation of animal magnetism and called it absurd. However, he supported the idea of the power of the imagination and was 'disposed to attribute their recovery to the vigorous concurrence of the will in the action of the medicine' (Runes, 1947). The importance of expectation and imagination are clear indicators of success, just as they are in today's hypnobirthing programmes.

Discredited in France, Mesmer travelled to England and through Europe for some years before settling down in Meersburg, Germany, where he practised as a physician until he died in 1815, aged 80. Popularity for Mesmer declined following the two Royal Commissions, although animal magnetism, or mesmerism, continued to be practised in Europe and America. In 1825 the French Academy of Medicine held another commission of inquiry which, after 5 years, issued a favourable report. The Academy chose not to publish this report and a further commission published an unfavourable report in 1837.

Artificial somnambulism and post-hypnotic suggestion

The Marquis de Puysegur (1751–1825) was a member of the French aristocracy and studied mesmerism. He believed that Mesmer's methods involving the induction of fits or convulsions in some patients would be therapeutically unworkable, and adopted a gentler technique. Puysegur used the peasants who lived in and around his chateau to study the techniques and effects of mesmerism. One of these early patients was a young man called Victor Race. Puysegur tied the young man to a 'magnetised' tree and, whilst he was making magnetic passes over Race's head, he noticed that the patient appeared to enter a sleep-like state, which he called *artificial somnambulism*. Puysegur would make suggestions to his patients and discovered that not only would they follow these suggestions during this trance state but, when told that when they awoke they would touch their knee, the subject would do so without remembering that this suggestion had been made. This is known as a post-hypnotic suggestion and can be used to prepare clients for subsequent sessions. For example, a suggestion could be made that each time that they practise hypnosis, the woman will find it easier and easier to achieve the level of relaxation that she desires, for a calmer, more comfortable birthing experience.

Surgery without anaesthetics

James Esdaile was a surgeon in the East India Company working in Hooghly, Bengal for almost a decade from 1845. He successfully used his own version of mesmerism to induce a very deep trance state that allowed him to operate painlessly on patients, without the use of anaesthetics. In his book *Mesmerism in India and its Practical Application in Surgery and Medicine*, Esdaile describes his methods and results (1851). In an 8-month period he successfully, and painlessly, operated on 73 patients. The operations included the removal of tumours, cataract operations and even limb amputations. Over a period of 10 years, Esdaile operated on hundreds of patients using mesmerism. Around one-third of his patients felt no pain at all; one-third of patients were aware of something happening and, although on occasion they showed physical signs of pain, they had no memory of it afterwards. One-third never reached a suitably deep trance state for surgery to be undertaken. The chief drawback was the length of time required to get the patient into a deep enough trance to operate. This would take 2 to 3 hours a day for several days and in some cases as long as a week before the patient was ready. The popularity of mesmerism was growing, but in 1846 a Boston dentist by the name of William Thomas Green Morton successfully used sulphuric ether for the first time. Although this was an important advance in anaesthetics, the patient he operated on had asked to be mesmerised!

This early exploratory process has informed current hypnobirth practice. The level of relaxation required for birth can take weeks to achieve. The self-hypnosis techniques taught in hypnobirth require practice for mothers to become easily and deeply relaxed, which is why practice is so important.

A committee was set up by the Bengal Government to examine Esdaile's claims, a report of which can be found in the *Edinburgh Medical & Surgical Journal* entitled the 'Calcutta Report on Mesmerized Patients' (Hume, 1847). It supported his findings. In the same journal James Braid commented on the work of Esdaile. Although they had both performed surgical operations on patients in a deep trance state, they differed in the theory. Braid writes, 'In theory I entirely differ from Dr Esdaile. He is a mesmerist, – that is, he believes in the transmission of some peculiar occult influence from the operator to the patient, as the cause of the subsequent phenomena' (Braid, 1847).

Hypnotism

James Braid, MRCSE was a Scottish physician living and working in Manchester in the nineteenth century. Braid had read and heard about mesmerism but was unconvinced of its efficacy. He considered it to be a system of collusion or delusion. The first time that Braid had the opportunity to see a demonstration of animal magnetism was in November 1841, when Charles Lafontaine, a French mesmerist, visited Manchester.

Over the next few days, Braid went to several demonstrations given by Lafontaine and was intrigued by the subject's inability to open his eyes. Braid was sure that there was a physiological reason for this and conducted some experiments of his own. Braid discovered that, by getting the subject to stare at a fixed point in such a way as to strain the eyes and the eyelids, a hypnotic state could be induced quickly. This first discovery led him to experiment further. The mesmerists had been severely criticised for their lack of robust research, so Braid meticulously recorded his methodology and findings, in order to provide the data from which he drew his conclusions. Before sharing his findings with his peers, Braid sent his work to the most sceptical members of the scientific community for their scrutiny.

In 1843 Braid published an exposition of his views and findings: *Neurypnology; or, the Rationale of Nervous Sleep*. Originally Braid called his new treatment

Neurypnology, which he later shortened to hypnotism. Braid is generally attributed with having coined the term hypnotism; he was, indeed, the first person to explain how hypnosis works based on hundreds of hours of research with different patients with a wide range of conditions and diseases.

Although Braid believed he was making a new discovery, he later went on to investigate the practices of 'Hindoos and Magi of Persia' and found that they had been using almost identical self-hypnosis techniques 'for ages before the Christian era – most probably from the earliest times' (Braid, 1852).

Braid also discovered that no one can be hypnotised unless they want to be, unlike the mesmerists who claimed that they 'had the power to overmaster patients irresistibly, even whilst at a distance' (Braid, 1899).

Over the following decade Braid extensively researched the effects on his patients and, in 1852, in his book, *Magic, Witchcraft, Animal Magnetism, Hypnotism and Electro-Biology*, he wrote:

> the origin and essence of the hypnotic condition, is the induction of a habit of abstraction or mental concentration, in which, as in reverie or spontaneous abstraction, the powers of the mind are so much engrossed with a single idea or train of thought as to render the individual unconscious of, or indifferently conscious to, all other ideas, impressions or trains of thought.

Although Braid knew absolutely that hypnosis is not sleep, the legacy of his original description stays with us now. The idea has been perpetuated by stage hypnotists who encourage the notion that their subject is in a deep sleep and under their control.

These are the beginnings of hypnosis as we understand it today. Of course since then techniques have been both refined and expanded. The following are some definitions given by people who have been influential in the field of hypnosis.

> I define hypnotism as the induction of a peculiar psychical condition which increases the susceptibility to suggestion.
>
> *(Bernheim, 1884)*

Bernheim was a nineteenth-century physician and professor at the University of Nancy. Sigmund Freud was a pupil of Bernheim's, and from his teachings psychoanalysis would emerge.

> [T]he hypnotic trance is a state of heightened susceptibility to suggestion.
>
> *(Hull, 1933)*

Hull was a psychologist and one of the first to empirically study hypnosis; he published the results of his rigorous studies in his book *Hypnosis and Suggestibility*.

> The hypnotic trance may be defined, for purposes of conceptualisation, as a state of increased awareness and responsiveness to ideas.
>
> *(Erikson, 1958)*

Erikson was a psychiatrist who specialised in medical hypnosis. He was the founder of the American Society for Clinical Hypnosis and was renowned for his approach to the unconscious mind. Erikson believed that a person's unconscious held all the solutions necessary to effect a change. He used a less direct form of hypnosis, something more conversational and subtle which relied more on rapport and trust. This works very well with hypnobirth, where a woman is working with her birthing partner and often with a midwife whom she has only just met. The gentle, yet powerful, techniques lend themselves to building rapport which can lead to deep relaxation.

> Hypnosis is a state of mind in which the critical faculty of the human is bypassed, and selective thinking established.
>
> *(Elman, 1964)*

Elman was another very important influence in hypnosis and developed a quick induction technique that is perfect for deep relaxation, and one that is often used by hypnobirthing couples. Dave Elman was born in 1900 and is considered to be one of the greatest hypnotists of all time. Elman's first experience of hypnosis being used for pain relief was when he was 8 years old. His father was dying of cancer and in a great deal of pain when a hypnotist used hypnosis to lessen the pain, which allowed him to play with Dave one more time. As a result, Elman was inspired to research hypnosis and its effects on pain.

Elman toured with vaudeville groups as a musician, comedian and stage hypnotist. By the age of 12, Elman's research had led him to develop his quick induction technique for use on stage. Vaudeville acts that were slow were considered boring and did not last. However, it was several decades later that Elman realised the significance of his fast induction technique and its uses in the field of medicine. During the remainder of his career, Elman trained many doctors and dentists how to use his rapid induction technique (Connelly, 2015).

What does hypnosis feel like?

Hypnosis feels like being relaxed, and this is definitely an important goal in hypnobirth. However, hypnosis is also about sharply focused attention and peak concentration. It can be used to enhance a particular mental resource or attitude. A hypnobirthing mother will use hypnosis in a variety of ways: for relaxation, to allow her muscles to work naturally during labour; for focused attention, to reduce peripheral distraction; and to build confidence during her pregnancy which, when combined with excellent antenatal education, will empower her and her birthing partner.

Hypnosis is a brain wave rhythm; it is a completely natural state of mind that is experienced throughout the day. It is like day dreaming or meditating. Many people have experienced hypnosis when doing a routine task, which will allow them to focus their attention on an unrelated topic. This often occurs when driving a familiar route and the driver suddenly realises that they are much further along their journey than they expected. It occurs when deeply engrossed in a book or a piece of music, to the extent that the reader, or listener, is unaware of other people, or sounds, around them.

The lovely floaty feeling just as you fall asleep is called hypnagogic; and as you begin to wake up is known as hypnapompic. 'Suggestibility seems to be one of the most predominant features of hypnogogia' (Mavromatis, 1987), which means that, when couples listen to the CD whilst falling asleep, the suggestions can be easily absorbed and accepted.

Myths and misconceptions

From before the times of the mesmerists, hypnosis has been thought of as something mystical and even magical, and this mystique has remained to some extent. This idea has been perpetuated by the media and by stage hypnotists for the entertainment of their audiences. In a clinical setting it is important to dispel the myths and misconceptions that abound.

Many people believe that hypnosis is something that is done to them. When people think of hypnosis, they generally think of a hypnotist and their subject, or patient; this might be in a one-to-one therapeutic environment or stage hypnosis for entertainment purposes. In a clinical setting, the hypnotist is a facilitator who makes suggestions that the client can accept and then begin to make the changes that he or she chooses. In an entertainment setting, the subject is a willing participant who has been given permission to do something funny, or daft, without having to take any responsibility for their behaviour.

A good hypnobirth teacher, who can provide excellent antenatal information, will share tried and tested hypnosis techniques, which the couples will learn, practise and become experts in, for themselves. When a person switches from being a passive to an active participant, hypnosis and hypnobirth techniques become more effective, allowing couples to have the best experience, no matter what situations may arise.

When people first experience hypnosis, they often think that nothing is happening. This is because they believe that they will fall asleep, or be unconscious, and will be unable to hear anything. The opposite is true, they will be aware of everything going on around them. Sometimes people feel as if their awareness is expanding; at other times they will become so focused on a script or a breathing technique that everything else around them fades away; this is completely normal.

Historically hypnosis has been referred to as a trance, which is appropriate when made clear that it resembles day dreaming, or focused concentration. It was believed that an altered state of consciousness was required for successful hypnosis, but extensive research shows that this is not the case, and this hypothesis has been rejected by most researchers (Kirsch and Lynn, 1995). The idea of being 'put into a trance' can make people anxious and inhibit their experience of hypnosis until they realise that they are in control.

People may be afraid about losing control and doing something daft or sharing their deepest, darkest secrets. It is important to remember that a hypnotist cannot make someone do something against their will. If a suggestion is made which conflicts with a client's morals or ethics, they will either ignore it or they might adapt it to suit their beliefs. So if I were to tell a client in hypnosis that at the end of the session they go and rob a bank, and bring me all the money, they will ignore this suggestion; at least, they have so far!

When a person first experiences hypnosis, they are likely to feel some scepticism, especially if they believe that it was something that was going to be done to them. It may help them to have a more positive experience if they suspend their scepticism and simply go with the ideas that are being suggested. Hypnobirth courses use visualisation scripts that offer an opportunity to become actively involved in the process. They give clients a visual cue to their level of suggestibility, which can help them to understand how they may be affected by the language used during their pregnancy, and labour.

Sometimes people worry that they could get stuck in hypnosis. However, hypnosis is a normal brainwave rhythm between being fully alert and asleep, which means that they will either become fully alert at the end of their practice, or they may fall asleep, especially when they are practising the relaxation techniques at bedtime.

Hypnosis and the brain

With the ability to measure, hypnosis has moved from the magical realms into the scientific. The work done by neuroscientists, especially with brain imaging, has helped to explain the physiology of hypnosis and the brain, and that hypnosis is a function of the brain as well as of the mind.

Post-hypnotic suggestion and the Stroop test

In 2006, Raz *et al.* published a paper entitled 'Neuroimaging and Genetic Associations of Attentional and Hypnotic Processes', in which they describe how 'Brain imaging has forged an impressive link between psychology and neuroscience'. During their research they used the Stroop test (Stroop, 1935). The classic Stroop test requires experienced readers to identify the colour of the ink of the word that is displayed. There are three elements in the test:

1. the name of a colour that is the same as the colour of the ink, e.g. GREEN written in green ink;
2. the name of a colour that is different from the colour of the ink, e.g. GREEN written in purple ink;
3. A control word, that is not a colour, e.g. TABLE written in blue ink.

It takes longer to identify the colour of the ink, and often has more errors, when the colour of the ink is different from the name of the colour (2), compared with when the word and colour of the ink matches (1), or when seeing a control word (3). The reason for the delay, and for the extra errors, is because the brain will read the word more quickly than it can identify the colour of the ink. When there is no conflict, the brain simply ignores the word.

This exercise is often seen in brain-training games, and by concentrating and plenty of practice it is possible to improve the accuracy of the test; however, experienced readers will automatically access the meaning of the word, which can delay the identification of the colour of the ink, when the word and colour are in conflict. This delay is known as the Stroop Interference Effect.

In the test, subjects were introduced to the following post-hypnotic suggestion: that although the words were written in English, the suggestion was made that they were written in a foreign language that the test subjects could not understand. This time, the brain ignored the words, and even when there was a conflict between the word and the colour (2), the subject identified the colour more quickly, and accurately, more often.

Hypnobirth uses many post-hypnotic suggestions in the scripts, to promote confidence in the woman's ability to deeply relax and birth her baby with ease.

Visualisation enhances peak performance

Mental training through meditation can change the neuroplasticity of the brain (Davidson and Lutz, 2008). Neuroplasticity refers to the brain's ability to restructure itself after training or practice. In 1987, the fourteenth Dalai Lama, Tenzin Gyatso, started the Mind and Life Institute with neuroscientist Francisco Varela, and entrepreneur and lawyer, Adam Engle. 'The Mind and Life Institute is a non-profit organisation committed to building a scientific understanding of the mind as a way to help reduce suffering and promote human flourishing' (Mind and Life Institute, 2015). In 1987, the first 'dialogue' was held, which discussed Buddhism and the Cognitive Sciences. The dialogue series was created to bridge the gap between scientists and well-refined contemplative disciplines, in order to enhance human well-being. Amongst the topics discussed, 'How the brain works' is a recurring theme.

Dr Richard J. Davidson, a neuroscientist at the Waisman Laboratory for Brain Imaging and Behaviour at the University of Wisconsin-Madison, has been a regular participant in the dialogue series. Davidson has been interested in meditation since the early 1970s, when he was a post-graduate student at Harvard, and, although he conducted a few studies on the attentional abilities of people who meditated regularly, it was not until 1992 that he began to focus more on this subject. Davidson knew of the Dalai Lama's interest in science, and wrote to ask if he could study some of Tibetan Buddhism's expert meditators. Davidson wanted to test the lasting effect on the brain as a result of thousands of hours of meditating, to see whether changes were perceptible, even when the person was not meditating. The Dalai Lama had recently become interested in neuroscience and gave his

TABLE 2.1 Brain wave oscillations

Super concentration	Gamma	25–70Hz
Fully conscious awareness	Beta	13–30Hz
Light relaxation	Alpha	8–13Hz
Deep relaxation	Theta	4–8Hz
Sleep	Delta	0.1–4Hz

permission. Unfortunately the meditators were not so keen; they had chosen a life of solitude in the hills around Dharamsala and they all declined Davidson's invitation (Davidson and Begley, 2012; Begley, 2008).

It was not until 2001, in response to a request from the Dalai Lama, that French-born Matthieu Ricard offered to take part, and the planned research would begin. Ricard was born in 1946, had a PhD in molecular biology and had been a Tibetan Buddhist monk since his early twenties. Eventually, Davidson found eight monks with between 10,000 and 50,000 hours of meditation experience willing to take part in his study and a control group of Madison undergraduates who were given a quick course in meditation (Lutz *et al.*, 2004).

The study showed that the monks had greater levels of gamma oscillations, the rhythms that are present with higher levels of focus and organisation, than the control group (Davidson and Lutz, 2008).

Hypnosis occurs during both alpha and theta brain waves, depending on the depth of relaxation. Gamma waves are thought to link activity in all parts of the brain. If we think of brain waves as the musical notes of an orchestra, when we listen to the instruments being tuned this would be the brain working in an uncoordinated way. Gamma waves would be the conductor who coordinates the individual notes, and together they create beautiful music.

Everyone has gamma waves in varying levels; more gamma waves means greater concentration; people with learning disabilities have fewer gamma waves. High achievers in all fields including athletes, musicians and other performers show high levels of both alpha and gamma waves during peak performance activity. Hypnosis has been used by these groups for decades to enhance and hone their skills. Just as with any activity, the more we focus and practise, the better we become. The same is true with hypnobirthing couples.

When the myths are debunked and hypnosis is treated collaboratively, people are able to lose any scepticism and anxiety that they may have, so that they can grow in confidence and reap the benefits of the techniques that they learn.

Bibliography

Begley, S. (2008). *Train your mind, change your brain*. New York: Ballantine Books.
Bernheim, H. (1884). *Hypnosis and suggestion in psychotherapy*. Paris: Octave Doin.
Binet, A. and Féré, C. (1888). *Animal magnetism*. New York: D. Appleton & Co.
Braid, J. (1899). *Braid on hypnotism. Neurypnology*. London: George Redway.

Braid, J. (1852). *Magic, witchcraft, animal magnetism, hypnotism and electro-biology.* London: John Churchill.

Braid, J. (1847). Facts and observations as to the relative value of mesmeric and hypnotic coma, and ethereal narcotism, for the mitigation or entire prevention of pain during surgical operations. *The Edinburgh Medical and Surgical Journal*, 588–592.

Braid, J. (1843). *Neurypnology; or, the rationale of nervous sleep considered in relation with animal magnetism.* London and Edinburgh: John Churchill and Adam & Charles Black.

Cilliers, L. and Retief, F. (2013). Dream healing in Asclepieia in the Mediterranean. In S. Oberhelman, *Dreams, healing, and medicine in Greece: From antiquity to the present.* Ashgate e-Book.

Colgan, R. (2012). *Advice to the healer: On the art of healing.* New York, Heidelberg, Dordrecht, London: Springer Science+Business Media.

Connelly, T. (2015). Heroes of Hypnosis – Dave Elman. hypnosis-online.co.uk: http://www.hypnosis-online.co.uk/elmanhypnotherapy.htm. Retrieved September 22nd 2015.

Davidson, R. and Begley, S. (2012). *The emotional life of your brain.* New York: Hudson Street Press.

Davidson, R. and Lutz, A. (2008). Buddha's brain: Neuroplasticity and meditation. *IEEE Signal Process Magazine*, 25(1), 171–174.

Ellenberger, H. F. (1981). *The discovery of the unconscious. The history and evolution of dynamic psychiatry.* New York: Perseus Books Group.

Elman, D. (1964). *Hypnotherapy.* London: Westwood Publishing.

Erickson, M. (1958). Naturalistic techniques of hypnosis. *American Journal of Clinical Hypnosis*, 1, 3–8.

Esdaile, J. (1851). *Mesmerism in India and its practical application in surgery and medicine.* New York: Silus Andrus & Son.

Gauld, A. (1992). *A history of hypnotism.* Cambridge, New York: Cambridge University Press.

Hull, C. (1933). *Hypnosis and suggestibility.* New York and London: D. Appleton-Century-Crofts.

Hume, J. (1847). Calcutta report on mesmerized patients. *The Edinburgh Medical and Surgical Journal*, 581–588.

Kirsch, I. and Lynn, S. J. (1997). Hypnotic involuntariness and the automaticity of everyday life. *American Journal of Clinical Hypnosis*, 40, 329–348.

Kirsch, I. and Lynn, S. (1995). The altered state of hypnosis: Changes in the theoretical landscape. *American Psychologist*, 50, 846–858.

Lanska, D. and Lanska, J. (2007). Franz Anton Mesmer and the rise and fall of animal magnetism: Dramatic cures, controversy, and ultimately a triumph for the scientific method. In H. S. Whitaker, *Brain, mind and medicine: Essays in eighteenth-century neuroscience* (pp. 301–320). New York: Springer U.S.

Lilienfield, S., Lynn, S., Namy, L., Woolf, I., Jamieson, G., Marks, A. and Slaughter, V. (2014). *Psychology, from inquiry to understanding.* Melbourne: Pearson Australia.

Lutz, A., Greischar, L., Rawlings, N., Ricard, M. and Davidson, R. (2004). Long-term meditators self-induce high-amplitude gamma synchrony during mental practice. *Proceedings of the National Academy of Sciences*, (101), 16369–16373.

Mavromatis, A. (1987). *Hypnagogia: The unique state of consciousness between wakefulness and sleep.* London: Routledge and Kegan Paul.

Mind and Life Institute (2015). mindandlife.org: https://www.mindandlife.org/mission. Retrieved September 23rd 2015.

Osler, W. (2004). *The evolution of modern medicine.* Whitefish, Montana: Kessinger Publishing.

Osler, W. (1892). *The principles and practice of medicine.* Edinburgh and London: Young J. Pentland.

Raz, A., Fan, J. and Posner, M. (2006). Neuroimaging and genetic associations of attentional and hypnotic processes. *Journal of Physiology*, Paris, 483–491.

Runes, D. (1947). *The selected writings of Benjamin Rush*. Unknown: Philosophical Library.

Rush, B. (1812). *Medical enquiries and observations, upon the diseases of the mind*. Philadelphia: Kimber & Richardson.

Spiegel, H. (1981). Hypnosis: Myth and reality. *Psychiatric Annals*, 11(305), 711–716.

Spiegel, H. and Spiegel, D. (1978). *Trance and treatment: Clinical uses of hypnosis* (2nd edn). Arlington, Virginia: American Psychiatric Publishing.

Stroop, J. (1935). Studies of interference in serial verbal reactions. *Journal of Experiments Psychology*, 18, 643–661.

3

WHY HYPNOBIRTH?

Birth in Western society is often portrayed as painful and terrifying (Mongan, 2007). The undercurrent in society suggests that birth is a medical event and best performed in the hospital, confirming a technocratic belief that birth is inherently unsafe (Davis-Floyd, 1992). The National Institute for Health and Care Excellence (NICE, 2012) places childbirth under the heading of 'condition and disease'.

These beliefs can result in women approaching birth fearfully and with little confidence. The vast majority of the pregnant population is well informed, sophisticated and information hungry. With sources of knowledge available in many formats, it is almost impossible to remain uninvolved. Just switching on the television may result in viewing someone else's labour. Pregnancy information is available in the form of blogs, forums, documentaries, apps and websites. These can be a great source of information, but much of it is opinion based.

When women require more structured information, they begin to research what is on offer in their area. Often the choice is NHS-based classes or private classes such as the NCT. Some might say that NHS classes are process driven, focusing on the anatomy of birth and the pharmacology of pain. NCT classes offer a wider, holistic approach. Traditionally NHS classes are short on time, with classes varying widely across the country. Most are full to capacity, as spaces are few and hospitals struggle to fulfil the need. NCT classes offer enough hours to discuss diverse topics, such as changing relationships and post-natal issues. They offer small groups that encourage interaction and socialisation. Hypnobirth classes have closed the gap between the two, offering the anatomy and physiology, evidence-based education and a holistic approach to pain management.

Hypnobirth, the 'brand', began in America where the increased medicalisation of birth has risen exponentially. It would appear that hypnobirth has gone some way to redressing the balance. Statistics for 2005–2010 provided by the Hypno-Birthing Institute gave a figure of 23 per cent epidural rate for hypnobirthers compared with the national average of 71 per cent (Dolce, 2010). When discussing hypnobirth and its effect, many studies look to epidural use as a point of reference. The use of epidural analgesia can be difficult to assess. Not all epidurals are effective, and many women are unaware that there is any failure rate. If the epidural is seen by the woman as something to enable her to cope, something she is pinning her hopes on, and then it is ineffective, where else is there to go? Sara Wickham explains that 'pain and pain relief are subjective and people have different expectations, the definition of "success" will vary between people, including researchers. To put it into research terms, there is no universal outcome measure for this'.

Women need a full range of coping skills for birth. The failure rate for epidural is small, and it is difficult to assess 'failure'. Wickham goes on to discuss: 'Does an epidural have to remove every last smidgen of sensation to be successful, or is it still a success if it removes 90 per cent of pain but the woman is OK with that?' (Wickham, 2014).

The best data suggest a failure rate of 23 per cent (Thangamuthu *et al.*, 2013). This still involves some uncertainties, but it is clearly difficult to assess definitive figures.

All pharmacological methods of pain relief have limitations and well recognised complications associated with their use. Whenever there is a reliance on sources that are external, there must be preparation for variation. An epidural can be absolutely appropriate for some women. However the epidural 'solution' often means that a woman must behave passively during a potentially dynamic event. A medicalised labour and birth inhibits the production of hormones. It does not allow the woman to experience the profound satisfaction of the birthing experience. The wish to repeat the experience is dramatically reduced and bonding can be affected. The labour experience becomes a traumatic event that is retold – thus compounding the horror stories of birth.

Reducing or eliminating the need for analgesia in labour will reduce the incidence of complications and potentially improve the childbirth experience. An improved childbirth experience can have an impact on recovery, the bonding experience, breastfeeding, post-natal depression, and self-esteem.

If hypnosis for birth can offer the benefit of reducing pain without the associated complications of pharmacological analgesia, then logic tells us that this is an area worthy of further exploration. However hypnobirth offers a multifaceted range of benefits, and to narrow the focus to epidural use is limiting. Most research into the area of hypnobirth has traditionally focused on the effects of the hypnosis on birth outcomes. Many studies use a quantitative approach and focus on outcomes such as reducing the need for analgesia during labour and length of labour.

The research

The 2015 SHIP trial (Self-hypnosis for intrapartum pain management in pregnant nulliparous women) is the largest randomised controlled trial undertaken in the UK to date. This took place across three NHS Trusts in 2011–2013, using seven sites and 672 participants. A total of 337 were randomly allocated to the intervention group receiving hypnosis alongside usual NHS care and 335 to the control group receiving usual NHS care alone. The hypnosis intervention consisted of two 90-minute hypnosis sessions at 32 weeks' and 35 weeks' gestation. Participants also received a relaxation CD for practice at home. In contrast, most standard hypnobirth courses are between 10 and 12 hours. The contact with participants is four or five sessions, and practice with a relaxation CD is encouraged daily. The SHIP trial results revealed a total of 39.4 per cent of practice logs were returned, which equated to an average of three practice sessions a week. Birth companions were reported to practise with participants for 24.5 per cent of the sessions. The report states:

> It is logical to assume that women who were most likely to undertake regular practice were over-represented among those who returned their logs. Conservatively, therefore, fidelity to the protocol was likely to be lower over the whole intervention group.
>
> *(Downe et al., 2015)*

We hear from teachers and couples that the value of the hypnobirth course is the involvement of the birth partner. We also know that the effectiveness of hypnosis relies on repetition and practice. The SHIP trial concluded that self-hypnosis training did not affect the rates of epidural anaesthesia or most of the intrapartum and psychosocial variables tested for in the study. The impact of women's anxiety and fear about childbirth needs further investigation. Interestingly the limitations of the study include the non-hypnosis control group using hypnosis in labour: 'the ability of the study to address the objectives is limited by the fact that approximately 10 per cent of the control group reported using self-hypnosis in labour'. It is a testament to the popularity of hypnobirth that women selected for the control group independently sought hypnosis as childbirth preparation.

A Cochrane Review published in 2012 included seven trials that randomised 1,213 women to hypnosis or to control groups receiving: standard childbirth preparation; usual care; a relaxation tape combined with relaxation practice in antenatal classes; or supportive counselling or supportive psychotherapy. There were no significant differences between women in the hypnosis group and those in the control group in terms of additional use of drugs for pain management. Small, single trials reported that hypnosis reduced pain intensity, shortened the length of labour and reduced the number of women who stayed in hospital for more than 2 days after their baby was born, compared with women who received relaxation training or supportive counselling. The Cochrane Review concluded that 'Hypnosis may help relieve pain in labour but research so far conducted has not conclusively shown benefit' (Madden *et al.*, 2012).

The Cochrane Review comments on the timing of the hypnosis intervention as significant. Subgroup analysis indicated that there was an interaction between the trimester that hypnosis commenced and use of pharmacological analgesia. The use of pharmacological analgesia appeared to be lower when the intervention began in the second or third trimester.

An Australian, single-centred, randomised controlled trial, the HATCh Trial (Cyna *et al.*, 2006a), found hypnosis to reduce the need for epidural anaesthesia in 77 primigravid and multiparous women. Of the primigravid women, 36 per cent experienced birth without epidural, compared with 53 per cent of the control group. Of the multiparous women, 67 per cent, compared with 54 per cent of the control group, gave birth without epidural anaesthesia. The hypnosis group had received three sessions of hypnosis training antenatally. Each session was 60 minutes long, in groups of 5–10 women. Participants in the hypnosis group were compared with a control group of 3,249 women, matched for parity and gestational age, who had received standard medical care. Information on the control group was collected from retrospective chart data. Limitations of the study were that the women had 'self-selected' and were all interested in hypnosis. The study looked only at epidural use and not other forms of pharmacological pain management.

Landolt and Milling (2011) performed a methodological review using 13 studies. They compared hypnosis versus standard medical care; hypnosis versus supportive counselling; hypnosis versus Lamaze; and hypnosis versus childbirth education classes. Three studies comparing hypnosis with supportive counselling and childbirth education classes failed to show a positive effect for hypnosis on at least one indicator of pain.

Ten studies have supported hypnosis as a positive intervention for reducing epidural use and pain experience. Three studies (Jenkins and Pritchard, 1993; Davidson, 1962; and Harmon *et al.*, 1990) reported significantly shorter labours. Of the 13 studies used, only three were published in the last 10 years (Cyna *et al.*, 2006b; VandeVusse *et al.*, 2007; Mehl-Madrona, 2004). Landolt and Milling's conclusion was that hypnosis outperformed standard care in reducing pain, but also reduced the length of first-stage labour and was associated with higher Apgar scores.

A large Danish quantitative study, inspired by the Australian HATCh Trial, looked at healthy primigravid women (Werner *et al.*, 2012). They compared three groups: a hypnosis group receiving three 1-hour lessons in self-hypnosis with additional CDs; a relaxation group receiving three 1-hour lessons in various relaxation methods and mindfulness with additional CDs; and a usual care group receiving ordinary antenatal care only. The conclusions were that there was no difference in use of epidural analgesia or in pain experience within all groups. This study invited 3,554 women to participate. The response rate was 1,222. The low participation rate would suggest that antenatal hypnosis is not commonplace in this particular area. It may suggest some reluctance and/or suspicion to become involved. Interestingly, of the hypnosis intervention group, only 85.2 per cent of women received the whole course. Within the relaxation group, 79.8 per cent of women received the whole course. However 100 per cent of women in all three groups received epidural information. It could suggest a strong bias towards pharmacological analgesia. A figure of 59 per cent of the women also participated in antenatal training given by private providers concurrently with the allocated treatment. Hypnosis training relies heavily on the use of positive language and a philosophy towards birth. If the woman is receiving two conflicting antenatal programmes, then it is reasonable to assume that the hypnosis training is diluted.

Many of the studies used hypnosis preparation for birth that lasted no longer than 3 hours. Most current hypnobirth courses offered in the UK span 10–12 hours. The limitation of using randomised controlled trials (RCTs) to evaluate hypnobirth is the lack of rich data in the results. There is little qualitative evidence to assess women's experience of using hypnosis for birth, and further research is needed in all areas.

Breuer (2000) discussed placebo effectiveness and suggested that patients must accept their role in their own health care and needed to feel that the practitioner was credible for the hypnosis to be successful. This is resonant with current hypnobirth courses on offer. It may be that, by taking responsibility for the birth and engaging in education, the women choosing to hypnobirth feel more in control and more empowered than those who do not.

What women say

There is very little published on the impact of hypnosis preparation antenatally and its effect on the way a woman feels about birth. The SHIP trial finds that women in the intervention group using hypnosis had a greater reduction in anxiety and fear levels than they expected, compared with those in the control group. There is a visible gap in the research into this area, which needs further investigation. It is notoriously difficult to evaluate a woman's experience in labour. There are so many variables, and no two women will experience birth in the same way. The timing of the hypnosis, the skill of the practitioner, the length of the hypnosis sessions, the amount of practice and the involvement of the birth partner all contribute to the outcome. With such variables it may be almost impossible to reduce the experience to statistical data.

Anecdotally, women report feeling more confident, better prepared and less fearful on completion of the hypnosis course. There is, however, no current qualitative research to support this. It is often the birth partner who seems to benefit equally from the hypnobirth course. They report feeling well prepared and confident, and are skilled birth supporters. Again the impact of an effective birth partner in labour, whether hypnobirthing or not, needs to be assessed.

With the promise of quicker labours, reduced need for pharmacological analgesia and higher vaginal birth rates, a hypnobirth course seems a very attractive option for many women. The Mongan method used in the USA talks widely about pain-free birth. This concept is so far removed from most women's perception of birth that discovering more is almost irresistible. It may be the promise of a pain-free birth that brings a woman to a hypnobirth class. It may be her birth partner. It is more often the friend who used the techniques with success. Many women and their partners, once they give birth using hypnosis, become a little evangelical about the programme.

As women seek to improve their knowledge and coping skills for labour, a hypnobirth course offers more than traditional antenatal classes.

BOX 3.1 ALEX'S STORY

Having already used similar techniques successfully on a fear-of-flying course, I knew that relaxation could be used to effectively alleviate fear and, at the very least, thought that hypnobirthing might help reduce anxiety in the run-up to the birth. I was realistic about its potential to manage pain but any relief would be a bonus! I knew a number of people who had tried hypnobirthing or similar techniques during their labour, albeit using books and/or CDs. All of them said it was worthwhile.

Before I embarked on the course, I had no fixed idea about the type of birth I wanted. I had little understanding of how labour might be affected by being at home versus being in hospital, what induction involved and how active birth or the use of a pool could help with the speed of delivery and pain. However, I was open minded about the different options available to me. The course (as opposed to the books and CD alone) empowered me to make my own decisions about my birth plan and labour, and gave me confidence that they would be respected by the midwives. Being a complete first-timer, I found the antenatal content just as useful as the practical exercises. I took a lot from understanding the biological process of pregnancy and birth and used it to inform my birth plan. By the end of the course, I was positively evangelical about natural birth and hypnobirthing.

References

Breuer, C. W. (2000). The use of hypnosis in a primary care setting. *CRNA: The Clinical Forum for Nurse Anesthetists*, 186–189.

Cyna, A. M., Andrew, M. I., Robinson, J. S., Crowther, C. A., Baghurst, P., Turnbull, D. and Whittle, C. (2006a, March 5th). Hypnosis antenatal training for childbirth (HATCh trial): A randomised controlled trial [NCT00282204]. BioMed Central Pregnancy and Childbirth: www.biomedcentral.com. Retrieved November 13th 2013.

Cyna, A. M., Andrew, M. I., Robinson, J. S., Crowther, C. A., Baghurst, P., Turnbull, D. and Whittle, C. (2006b). Antenatal self-hypnosis for labor and childbirth: A pilot study. *Anesthesia Intensive Care*, 464–469.

Davidson, J. A. (1962). An assessment of the value of hypnosis in pregnancy and labour. *British Medical Journal*, 951–953.

Davis-Floyd, R. (1992). *Birth as an American rite of passage* (1st edn). Los Angeles: University of California Press.

Dolce, K. (2010, November 6th). HypnoBirthing Institute: http://hypnobirthing.com/US_Outcomes_Summary_2010.pdf. Retrieved July 5th 2014.

Downe, S., Finlayson, K., Melvin, C., Spiby, H., Ali, S., Diggle, P., Gyte, G., Hinder, S., Miller, V., Slade, P., Trepel, D., Weeks, A., Whorwell, P. and Williamson, M. (2015). Self-hypnosis for intrapartum pain management in pregnant nulliparous women; a randomised control trial of clinical effectiveness. *British Journal of Obstetrics and Gynaecology*, 1226–1234.

Harmon, T. H., Hynan, M. and Tyre, T. (1990). Improved obstetric outcomes using hypnotic analgesia and skill mastery combined with childbirth education. *Journal of Consulting and Clinical Psychology*, 525–530.

Jenkins, M. W. and Pritchard, M. H. (1993). Hypnosis: Practical applications and theoretical considerations in normal labour. *British Journal of Obstetrics and Gynaecology*, 221–226.

Landolt, A. S. and Milling, L. S. (2011). The efficacy of hypnosis as an intervention for labor and delivery pain: A comprehensive methodological review. *Clinical Psychology Review*, 31, 1022–1031.

Madden, K., Middleton, P., Cyna, A. M., Matthewson, M. and Jones, L. (2012). Hypnosis for pain management during labour and childbirth. *Cochrane Database of Systematic Reviews*, (11), art. no: CD009356. doi: 10.1002/14651858.CD009356.pub2.

Mehl-Madrona, L. (2004). Hypnosis to facilitate uncomplicated birth. *American Journal of Clinical Hypnosis*, 299–312.

Mongan, M. (2007). *HypnoBirthing*. London: Souvenir Press.

NICE (2012). www.nice.org.uk/guidance. Retrieved December 3rd 2012.

Thangamuthu, A., Russell, I. F. and Purva, M. (2013). Epidural failure rate using a standardised definition. *International Journal of Obstetric Anesthesia*, 22(4), 310–315.

VandeVusse, L., Irland, J., Berner, M., Fuller, S. and Adams, D. (2007). Hypnosis for child birth: A retrospective comparitive analysis of outcomes in one obstetrician's practice. *American Journal of Clinical Hypnosis*, 109–119.

Werner, A., Uldbjerg, N., Zachariae, R., Rosen, G. and Nohr, E. (2012). Self-hypnosis for coping with labour pain: A randomised controlled trial. *British Journal of Obstetrics and Gynaecology*, 120, 346–353.

Wickham, S. (2014, March 31st). What is the success/failure rate of epidurals? sarawickham. com: www.sarawickham.com/questions-and-answers/what-is-the-successfailure-rate-of-epidurals. Retrieved June 3rd 2015.

4

THE NEOCORTEX IN LABOUR AND BIRTH HORMONES

Labour is unique in presenting a woman with stressors which can both benefit and detract from the experience. Labour stress has been shown to trigger and enhance adaptive responses in both mother and baby, which may contribute to the prevention of adverse labour outcomes such as fetal and/or maternal morbidity and mortality (Pirdel, 2009). If these adaptive responses are so crucial, it is wise to assume that undisturbed birth and physiological hormones are to be supported at all times. Uvnas-Moberg (2003) describes a woman's biological rhythms as connected. She suggests that the external environment dictates the internal environment.

A 2009 study into environmental stressors and pain perception concluded: 'Performance of routine diagnostic tests in hospitalized pregnant woman, provision of invasive medical care during labour process and a noisy and crowded environment all influence the mother's experience and perception of pain' (Pirdel, 2009).

Hospital birth and labour

Many women choose to birth in a hospital environment. Hospital birth is now the norm. The growth of hospitalisation for birth has been continuing since the 1960s and 1970s, two decades which saw the greatest expansion in hospital-building programmes and changes in the organisational structure of the NHS (Hunt, 1995). The declining homebirth rate suggests that women are not confident in birthing at home and view hospital as the safest option. When a woman does choose to home birth, the midwife is obliged to complete a risk assessment. The subtext for this conversation is that home birth is unsafe. Interestingly the same risk assessment is not performed for hospital birth. To be equitable, the implementation of a hospital birth form would be advantageous. This could risk assess the likelihood of infection, intervention, one-to-one care in labour and pain relief rates in hospital. For genuine choice of place of birth, many women need to be fully informed. Lemay

(2011) suggests that birth at home emphasises the importance of the process and not only the outcome.

For some women the only time that a visit to the hospital is required is when a friend or relative is poorly. The association with hospitals is one of sickness; Granshaw and Porter (1990) say that historically hospitals had been 'associated with pauperism and death'. In the reformation of the NHS post-Second World War, maternity services were hospitalised and free to all. Equal access to health care was on offer to all class systems for the first time, and many saw it as expert medical attention to which women were entitled. Home birth and midwives seemed to belong to a Victorian past and were connected to memories of poverty and deprivation (Hunt, 1995). Medicalisation and hospitalisation of birth led to a rise in research as large numbers of women were in one place. Along with mediatisation came social control and its relationship in midwifery (Hunt and Symonds, 1995).

Some women who choose a hospital birth have an inherent fear of hospitals. They instinctively feel more comfortable at home, but their rational mind is telling them that a hospital birth will be safer. This can cause real anxiety for some women.

Jodi says; 'As I walked into the hospital I reminded myself how the smell of the hospital resembled "life" and "healing"'. Jodi had worked hard on this affirmation, as by her own admission she was terrified of hospitals.

The anxiety in the move from home to hospital can increase the woman's stress hormones. These are catecholamines, epinephrine and norepinephrine. These hormones are released in response to stimuli and situations that the woman feels, sees or perceives as dangerous (Mongan, 2007). The stress reaction to an unfamiliar environment will provoke the fight-or-flight response. This is when the heart rate increases, breathing patterns become rapid and digestive systems slow as the body is preparing to flee the situation.

Oxytocin (again)

Much has been written about the role of oxytocin in labour. It is such an important element that it is worth a small recap.

Oxytocin is an essential hormone in all aspects of our lives. When forming relationships with other people, oxytocin plays a role. It enhances what is called 'social memory'. It can enable us to prefer certain individuals over another. When we meet someone with whom we feel a 'spark', it is oxytocin that we are feeling. In all female mammals it allows a mother to learn to recognise and prefer her own offspring. This is why babies produce their own oxytocin, to ensure the mother–baby bonding process.

Birth is dominated by a cocktail of hormones. When labour begins, the body releases oxytocin. This is received by oxytocin receptors in the uterus, which in turn produces the surge. The baby also produces oxytocin. Oxytocin is the power behind a labour. It produces and maintains the surge. This balance needs to be nurtured for labour to continue.

Oxytocin is stored in the anterior pituitary and is released in pulses every 3–5 minutes in early labour. This is a rhythm that the smooth muscles of the uterus respond to, and which establishes regular surges (Kresser, 2011). The spaces between the surges are just as important as the surges themselves. This is the time when the body adds another hormone – beta-endorphins. Endorphins are similar in effect to opiates, but naturally produced. They activate the mesocorticolimbic dopamine reward system, producing feelings of pleasure. Endorphins increase tolerance to pain and make the whole experience manageable.

BOX 4.1 JOY'S STORY

For me, as a musician, sound is very important. I chose to have sea and whale sounds during my labour as I felt this would help with feeling the 'surges' as waves, as well as being relaxing. My labour was quite long (19 hours or so), so we played other chosen music in between as well as listening to some hypno-birthing CDs. This definitely helped to stay focused. I found I was so relaxed that I could actually have conversations and even share a laugh with midwives or my partner without losing my calm state of mind. I also played on my small medieval harp quite a lot and when I was playing during my surges I didn't feel them in the same way at all. I even asked the midwife if they had stopped! I asked her if I should stop playing as I didn't want to slow things down! She said it was on the contrary – my surges were extremely powerful – they didn't change in their intensity when I was playing the harp, but I really didn't experience them in the same way. Playing the harp – whether it was the sounds, the vibrations on my body or the focus on playing – helped me go deeper into my body. Harps were used in ancient Greece to heal patients and now I know for sure that sound (even better if it's live) can change everything. It's just so incredibly important that a birthing woman can be silent or have the sounds and environment she chooses. I can see through my own experiences (after giving birth to two daughters) that the more relaxed, happy, confident and supported a woman can be during birth, the more likely there is to be an easy, gentle, natural birth. Hypnobirthing really works!

Oxytocin disruption

Oxytocin is an intimate hormone. It responds best to environmental and emotional influences. Couples produce large amounts of oxytocin when they make love. It is this that gives us a wonderful sense of fulfilment. To set the scene for romance and intimacy and to allow the oxytocin to peak, there may be some environmental influences that can encourage or discourage intimacy:

- Privacy – being able to relax is essential.
- Disruptions and disturbances interrupt the oxytocin flow.

- Peak oxytocin is more likely in an environment that is quiet, warm and softly lit.
- Oxytocin responds to our senses, so smells, music, good food and touch will all increase it.

The birth environment can affect oxytocin levels a great deal, and Niles Newton was writing about birth disturbances as early as 1960. She studied the effect of environment on the process and progress of labour in laboratory mice. Significantly more mice gave birth in a familiar covered nest box than those who were moved to a glass nest box. The addition of movement and observation to labour has proved detrimental. When a woman arrives in labour it can be the senses and instinct that overrule logic. She is birthing with her primal brain, the part that controls bodily functions, emotions and senses. This makes her receptive to the environment. Ask yourself this: when the labouring woman journeys from the car park into the Maternity area:

- Is it warm and welcoming?
- What will she smell?
- What will she hear?
- When she is greeted at the door, will it be by a stranger?
- When she is shown to the room, will the lights be on?
- Will there be somewhere comfortable to nest?
- Is there lovely food and drink available?
- Is there music?

Birth is instinctive, intimate and private. Yet the expectation is that women do it in a public building, with a stranger watching. We are realising the importance of maintaining the environment, and many maternity units have come a long way in adjusting the birth environment. They know the benefits of oxytocin release and the impact the environment has on it.

Midwives create and protect the environment for birth

Prepare in advance:

- darkness – dim the lights, dimmer switch, lamp
- change the smell – aromatherapy oils?
- music
- warm temperature
- bed to the side of the room
- alternative furniture – bean bag, birth ball, mats, rocking chair, birth stool
- privacy and quiet
- offer hydrotherapy-pool/bath/shower
- encourage nest building
- keep the pelvis upright and mobile

- consider rebozo
- massage
- breathing techniques.

BOX 4.2 RACHEL AND CHRIS'S STORY

At 8.15pm we arrived at the birth room and the midwife had also made her way in too. The welcoming birthing room and the midwife's presence made me feel instantly safe, calm and ready for birth. I believe my oxytocin levels at this point were high due to this perfect environment which enabled me to cancel out fear and anxiety. After an examination I discovered I was 9cm dilated. As I continued to breathe through the surges with some sacral massage from the midwife, the birthing pool was filled, the lights dimmed and the star projector created an amazing calming effect that filled the room. I felt safe and ready. Chris placed our LED candles around the space and the relaxation music used in class was played on my iPod.

The pool was both comforting and strangely euphoric, the warm water had such a soothing effect on my body I instantly let go of any tension. My surges were increasing steadily and I was approaching the next stage of labour. Both the midwife and Chris were supportive and attentive, but in a quiet and peaceful manner, remaining present, but allowing me to concentrate. It was at this point that I instinctively used the anchoring techniques learnt in class, using Chris's hand on my forehead as a point of strength and focus. The feeling of intense pressure, and a change in rhythm with regard to my surges, meant that the final stage was approaching, and my body felt as if it was starting to work harder to birth our baby. This feeling was strangely satisfying, and with the use of J breathing and a centred humming sound, I focused all my efforts down.

I never once believed that I was incapable of birthing our baby, and the use of any pain relief didn't even enter my head. I felt confident and determined with a deep sense of trust in my body and baby. Reaching forward and feeling my baby's head in the final stage of labour gave me that last rush of determination and strength. At 10.11pm Winnie Piper Grimsey arrived. Eased out of the water by Chris, with her eyes open and with a sense of serenity and wonder. Winnie was placed on my chest and lifted her head to focus on my face. This moment was intensely emotional and one I will never forget. I couldn't believe she was finally here, and I couldn't believe what I had achieved!

Synthetic oxytocin

The effect of synthetic oxytocin on the body is very different from naturally produced oxytocin.

In normal physiological labour, the baby's head on the cervix and placental and maternal hormonal changes result in early oxytocin production. In order for the woman to move into active labour, a rhythmic stimulus is needed to produce oxytocin on a constant and increasing basis. This stimulus is the intermittent sensation of labour. However, labour sensation can put the woman into an acute stress situation. The body reacts in the short term by producing the stress hormones catecholamines. These occur in peaks, in a pulsatile manner. Paradoxically, these increase the production of oxytocin and simultaneously produce endorphins and prolactin. This is the physiology of normal birth.

The rise of induction of labour sees the continuous use of prostaglandins and/or syntocinon. When hormones are added synthetically, the woman loses the pulsatile element of beta-endorphin production. Oxytocin is continuous and synthetic. Without the rhythmic peaks of natural labour, constant catecholamines are produced. Pain is increased and women often need additional analgesia (Buckley, 2009). Endorphins are reduced, and the feelings of fulfilment, well-being and euphoria present in an unmedicated birth are lost (Odent, 2009).

Concerns have been raised over the use of endogenous oxytocin and the long-term effects on the neonate. Odent (2009) states, 'Labor induction probably has life long consequences for the child.'

He suggests that induction and autism are an epidemic that have developed side by side. Children with autistic disorders show alterations in their oxytocin system, and this is linked to childbirth (Green et al., 2001). Kurth and Haussmann (2011) suggest that there may be a link between the use of syntocinon for induction and ADHD. Cerebral palsy quadriplegia was significantly more frequent after induction of labour (IOL) (45.5 per cent) compared with non-induced labour (8.0 per cent) (Elkamil et al., 2011). A Cochrane review examining the effectiveness of oxytocin on delay in first-stage labour concluded, 'The dilemma for obstetricians and mid-wives on labour wards is that a drug they have used for over 40 years to reduce the need for operative delivery has still not been proven to be effective in its original primary role' (Bugg et al., 2011).

It is apparent that the way in which birth begins needs further research, and the wider implications for future health are only now being discovered.

Catecholamines (CA)

Catecholamines are hormones epinephrine (adrenaline) and norepinephrine (nora-drenaline), usually produced in response to stress. During physiological labour, catecholamines gradually rise, peaking towards the end of first stage. Although we may think of these as stress hormones, they are perfectly designed to work on the final journey of opening, just before transition. They can be seen as emotion, distress, despair or aggression in the woman. It is important not to disturb the production of CA at this time. If left undisturbed, CA production often results in expulsive surges known as the fetal ejection reflex. Michel Odent, when talking about this stage of labour, suggests very little communication with the woman. He wants her to remain in her primal brain, connected to the hormones, and her body to work with them instinctively. When she feels anxious, desperate or emotional around the time of transition it is intuitive for the birth partner and/or the midwife to reassure, soothe and talk to her. Odent suggests that we keep all language to a minimum. In this way the neocortex is not stimulated, and the woman can move from first stage into the fetal ejection reflex.

> The passage towards the fetus ejection reflex is inhibited by any interference with the state of privacy. It does not occur if there is a birth attendant who behaves like a 'coach', or an observer, or a helper, or a guide, or a 'support' person.
>
> *(Odent, 2000)*

He goes on to say that the stimulation of language or bright lights will inhibit the fetal ejection reflex. All too often we do use language to ease the transition. We see it as a kindness, the need to reassure or instruct the woman during this time. In this way the woman experiences second-stage labour that may not have been necessary.

Catecholamines are an integral part of normal labour, and they must be in hormonal balance at all stages of labour for it to progress. If they rise too early in early labour as a result of disturbance, observation or perceived fear, they will lead to a slow or stalled labour. If the woman feels anxious or stressed, catecholamines are continuously produced and the body's production of oxytocin is inhibited. Labour is prolonged, latent phase extended, or the woman does not move into active labour. Later in labour they are needed for the fetal ejection reflex. If the natural CA levels have been blocked by analgesia in labour, then the fetal ejection reflex will be stalled and birth may be difficult.

The neocortex vs the primal brain

The neocortex is responsible for 'thinking behaviour'. This includes language and communication, social behaviour, problem solving, logic, spatial reasoning, conscious thought and sensory perception. Many women whom we meet in hypnobirth classes are well educated, ambitious, cerebral and work focused. Encouraging a reduction in the neocortex can be challenging. Often the word 'control' is used when women describe birth preparation. They come to hypnobirth looking to gain some control. We tell them that hypnobirth is a lesson in letting go of control! The best way to describe it is to liken it to lovemaking.

The aim/ultimate goal of lovemaking could be described as achieving an orgasm. For this to happen, there must be a physiological release of oxytocin. For oxytocin to happen a woman must feel safe, private, warm, intimate and relaxed. She must trust her partner. She must also switch off her neocortex. If she is constantly wondering about work, worrying about how she looks or if she is sweating or wondering if he can see her wobbly bits, she will never achieve the oxytocin release required for orgasm.

A reduction in neocortical activity is essential for a woman to labour successfully. Odent (2000) suggests that it is nature's way of protecting the woman from social and cultural conditioning. In normal circumstances she would find it difficult to express herself with primal noises. She might usually find the sweaty, swaying, rhythmic nature of labour unacceptable; the release of bodily fluids unpalatable. The reduction in neocortex activity places her 'in the zone' and she finds labour instinctive and primal. Odent goes on to say: 'Yet birth attendants, without any caution, constantly use language, the specifically human stimulant of the neocortex'.

Hypnobirth encourages the labouring woman to quieten the neocortex. She has practised for many weeks, and birth partners are well prepared for undisturbed birth. Hypnosis, as well as birth, takes place in the primal brain. All providers of care to labouring women should be aware of the need to reduce stimulation, especially language.

Top tips for neocortex reduction

- Keep the birthing room lights as low as possible.
- On arrival, gain as much information from the partner as possible before disturbing the woman.
- Read the birth plan.
- Once baseline observations are performed, gain consent to monitor baby and mother for the rest of labour. Document it; you can then perform observations without using language. This will feel very alien at first. Discuss with the parents the plan, and allow the woman to lead any conversation.
- Consider using a hypnobirth door sign. Give anyone else involved in the labour the heads up.

BOX 4.3 JOY AND JORGE'S BIRTH

In answer to the question 'What do you fear most?' (about birth), I suddenly realised that my answer was simple: 'Going into hospital'.

Being in a sterile, clinical environment with (potentially) bright lights, noise, machines bleeping, unfamiliar smells and interruptions as well as the possibility of being pushed into having (potentially) unnecessary interventions was my worst possible case scenario.

I was hoping for a home birth, but due to complications (obstetric cholestasis) I ended up in hospital at 3cm dilated. There was no emergency, no rush, so fortunately my partner and I had time to settle into our room in the high risk obstetric unit. Through our hypnobirthing course we had learnt to make a 'nest' and had brought our own blankets, pillows, battery operated candles, music, comfortable clothes and plenty of delicious snacks and drinks. This was of great importance in making me feel relaxed and able to focus on my baby and my body. One wall of the room was a giant photographic seascape and, even though there were the usual trappings of a hospital room, it made a huge difference to have such a beautiful wall (a piece of nature) in the room with us.

One of the midwives had witnessed a hypnobirth before and had also seen the film *Microbirth* so was totally convinced about the enormous benefits of having as natural a birth as possible. This was a huge relief. The other midwife reassured me she would make sure things were as quiet as possible and wouldn't use the words 'pain' or 'contraction'. They were wonderful. I was lucky to be able to have wireless monitoring (which should be offered as standard practice) so I could move around freely. I can't stress enough how important being able to be mobile is. Feeling free to move and get into any position I wanted as well as being able to make the room dark, quiet and as cosy as possible was absolutely essential to being able to birth without fear. Without that fear and tension in body or mind I could focus entirely on keeping relaxed and breathing my baby down. I knew the more relaxed I was, the greater the chance of a natural birth.

The one thing I would change about 'hypnobirthing' is the name itself! Many people think that it means you are not present, you remove yourself from the situation therefore don't feel anything. In my experience that is not the case at all. I have never felt more present, more relaxed and more confident that even if/when things got more challenging I knew I would be able to stay calm and breathe through it. Practising the hypnobirthing techniques was the key and completely transformed my experience of going into a frightening environment (hospital).

Bibliography

BirthchoiceUK (2012). Birthchoice UK. www.birthchoiceuk.com/Professionals/index.html. Retrieved November 18th 2012.

Buckley, S. (2009). *Gentle birth, gentle mothering* (1st edn). New York: Celestial Arts.

Bugg, G., Siddiqui, F. and Thornton, J. (2011, July 6th). Oxytocin versus no treatment or delayed treatment for slow progress in the first stage of spontaneous labour. *Cochrane Database of Systematic Reviews*. UK: John Wiley and Sons.

Elkamil, A. I., Andersen, G. L., Salvesen, K. Å., Skranes, J., Irgens, L. M. and Vik, T. (2011). Induction of labor and cerebral palsy: A population-based study in Norway. *Acta Obstetricia et Gynecologica Scandinavia*, 83–91.

Granshaw, L. and Porter, R. (1990). *The hospital in history* (1st edn). London: Routledge.

Green, L., Fein, D., Modahl, C., Feinstein, C., Waterhouse, L. and Morris, M. (2001). Oxytocin and autistic disorder: Alterations in peptides forms. *Biol Psychiatry*, 609–613.

Hunt, S. (1995). In O. Povey-Edmondson (ed.), *The social meaning of midwifery*. Houndmills: Macmillan Press.

Hunt, S. and Symonds, A. (1995). *The social meaning of midwifery*. Houndmills: Macmillan Press.

Kresser, C. (2011, August 3rd). Natural childbirth IV: The hormones of birth. http://chris kresser.com/natural-childbirth-iv-the-hormones-of-birth. Retrieved September 28th 2015.

Kurth, L. and Haussmann, R. (2011, July 10th). Perinatal Pitocin as an early ADHD biomarker: Neurodevelopmental risk? *Journal of Attention Disorders*, 15(5), 423–431.

Lemay, C. (2011). Reclaiming the meanings for birth, pain and risk within the home setting. In S. Donna (ed.), *Promoting normal birth. Research, reflections and guidelines* (pp. 170–179). Chester Le Street: Fresh Heart Publishing.

Mongan, M. (2007). *HypnoBirthing*. London: Souvenir Press.

Newton, N. F. D. (1966). Experimental inhibition of labor through environmental disturbances. *Obstet Gynecol*, 371–377.

Odent, M. (2009, September 4th). The midwives of Bethany Womens Healthcare. Birth Physiology: http://azmidwives.blogspot.co.uk. Retrieved March 19th 2013.

Odent, M. (2000). The second stage as a disruption of the fetus ejection reflex. *Midwifery Today*, 12.

Pirdel, M. P. L. (2009). Perceived environmental stressors and pain perception during labor among primiparous and multiparous women. *Journal of Reproductive Infertility*, 217–223.

Uvnas-Moberg, K. (2003). *The oxytocin factor. Tapping the hormone of calm, love and healing* (1st edn). London: Pinter and Martin.

5

THE POWER OF THE MIND

The conscious and the unconscious mind

In the early 1900s Sigmund Freud described the mind as an iceberg, which he divided into three levels, and assigned an estimate of the usage of each level:

- The conscious mind: 10 per cent – this would be the tip of the iceberg that is visible above the water and is used when we 'call something to mind'.
- The subconscious (or preconscious) mind: 10–15 per cent – this would be just below the surface of the water and holds all the information that can be accessed relatively easily.
- The unconscious mind: 75–80 per cent – this would be the largest part that is below the water and is not easily accessible (Freud, 1915).

Although popularity for Freud's psychoanalytical theories has waxed and waned, this model of the mind has withstood the test of time.

The conscious part of the mind, or the tip of the iceberg, is where we do all our logical thinking and it is responsible for decision making; it allows us to choose the direction of our focus. For many years it was believed that the conscious mind could remember seven, plus or minus two, randomly ordered pieces of information (Millar, 1956). These could be letters, numbers or words. More recent studies show this capacity to be limited to three to five separate items (Cowan, 2001), recognising that working memory capacity varies from one individual to another and changes with age (Cowan, 2005).

The subconscious part of the mind may be thought of as the store for information that can be retrieved easily. This would be information that is used every day, a telephone number perhaps, or the information that is taught in a hypnobirth class.

For the sake of simplicity, and because this book is about hypnobirth, the term 'conscious mind' will include the 'subconscious mind', as the information stored there is easily accessible, and they work closely together in our day-to-day thinking and activities.

The unconscious mind is by far the largest part of the mind and is where beliefs are stored, as are habits, emotions and feelings, as well as long-term memories. It is believed that all our experiences are stored in our long-term memory, although it is sometimes difficult to access it. 'It's in there somewhere, the problem is just getting to it,' Cowan said. 'Everything gets encoded into long-term memory almost immediately, but it gets encoded in a way that may not be distinct enough to be retrieved' (Cowan, 2005).

If the long-term memory stores everything, and the working memory can only process three or four things at a time, how does the unconscious part of the mind know which pieces of information to retrieve, or notice? How does it know what is important? Importance is decided by the conscious mind. For example, a person wants to buy a new car. After much research and deliberation they decide on the model and make that they wish to buy. They will then start to notice that particular car everywhere. Of course they have always been there, but the unconscious mind gave them little importance until the conscious mind told it to.

Leeman *et al.* (2003) suggest that a woman's confidence in her ability to cope with labour is the best predictor of pain during the first stage of labour. By focusing the mind on a calm, relaxed birth, the hypnobirthing couples give their minds the instruction to notice all the opportunities to help to make this a reality. By providing them with the knowledge and techniques, and with practice, they give themselves the best chance of achieving their desired outcome.

The unconscious mind is enormously powerful, it processes vast amounts of information all the time, as well as being responsible for running the autonomic systems. This means that, in a contest between the conscious and unconscious parts of the mind, no matter how much logic and willpower is used, the powerful unconscious part of the mind will eventually win. We can change our beliefs and habits with sufficient motivation, and with repetition of the new behaviour; however, hypnosis can assist the process, making the desired outcome much easier to achieve.

Habits and beliefs

When an action is repeated over and over again, it becomes a habit, and beliefs are created by repeating an idea. Beliefs, and habits, are often very powerful. Their power is linked to the strength of the emotion that was prevalent when the belief or habit was first formed, and they become more deeply embedded with every repetition.

The most enduring beliefs are formed when a person is young. They begin as an idea, a word, or a suggestion from someone influential in their lives; this might be a parent, a teacher, or a respected member of the community. These words or ideas can trigger strong feelings which, when repeated and reinforced, turn into beliefs. They can be positive or negative and will ultimately lead to success or failure.

A child growing up in an environment where they are constantly being criticised, told they are lazy or stupid, will take these beliefs into adulthood. A bad maths experience at school can result in the phrase 'I'm rubbish at maths', potentially a limiting, lifetime belief. A teenager viewing birth in a lesson at school can be left with an imprint that is difficult to change. It may only become relevant when she herself becomes pregnant, and wonders why she is fearful of birth.

When someone releases a limiting belief, it is important to replace it with a different thought. So, when working with couples, not only do we help them to let go of negative thoughts, we then replace them with positive thoughts, ideas and statements. Although a woman may have mixed feelings about pregnancy and birth, it is impossible for her to feel two opposite emotions at the same time – happiness versus anger, or relaxation versus tension or stress. The feeling with the strongest emotion attached to it will win.

The two wolves

You may have heard the story of the two wolves. An old Cherokee tells his grandson about the two wolves that are inside us all. One represents all the feelings and behaviours that we consider to be negative or bad: anger, envy, jealousy, greed and so on. The other wolf represents all that we consider to be positive and good: joy, peace, love, kindness, generosity, truth, compassion, etc. He explained to his grandson that these two wolves are in constant battle with one another. The grandson thought for a while and then asked, 'Which of these two wolves will win?' His grandfather replied, 'Whichever one you feed'.

The body is a 'robot'

What we focus on becomes reality: it begins with a thought which our body will turn into an action.

Dr Alvin M. Krasner was a world-renowned hypnotherapist, founding the American Institute of Hypnotherapy in 1981, and during his life he taught thousands of students all over the world. Krasner describes hypnosis as follows:

> I believe hypnosis to be a process which produces relaxation, distraction of the conscious mind, heightened suggestibility and increased awareness, allowing access to the subconscious mind through the imagination. It also produces the ability to experience thoughts and images as real.
>
> *(Krasner, 1990)*

In his book, *The Wizard Within* (1990), Krasner describes the unconscious mind as 'a powerful servo-mechanism, an uncritical, non judgemental computer. It accepts as true any suggestion that is allowed to bypass that critical factor of the conscious mind to make entrance to its system of memory banks.'

Krasner goes on to say that

> the body is only a robot acting and performing on command. The computer can be reprogrammed. The old data can be replaced. Through hypnosis, new beliefs and behaviours can be established. Remember: we always act and feel and perform according to what we imagine and believe to be true about ourselves and our surroundings.
>
> *(Krasner, 1990)*

Krasner named his book after the wizard in *The Wizard of Oz*, a childhood favourite of his. He liked to think of the mind as the 'wizard', and that every thought we have causes a physical response in the body.

If the body is a robot and the mind is the computer that runs it, where our mind leads, our body will follow. By the 1930s Dr Milton Erickson, an eminent psychiatrist, was renowned for his work in hypnosis. Erickson developed an induction technique that made the suggestion to the client that one hand was lighter than the other. The language used is very specific and the technique is quite complex, whilst sounding very simple. It demonstrated to the client how the unconscious mind will follow a suggestion resulting in one hand floating easily in the air whilst the other hand feels very heavy. Hypnobirth uses a simplified version of this technique to show couples how easily they can respond to simple suggestions. You might like to try this yourself or find a person, or a small group, to read it to:

Light arm/heavy arm exercise
[*Begin reading, and allow your listeners enough time to follow your instruction.*]
  Let's see how well you can use your imagination. Please stand comfortably. Let your arms just hang loosely at your sides. Good.
  Now raise both arms to shoulder height in front of you and allow both hands to hang downwards from the wrist. Now please turn your left palm upwards. And, when you're ready, you can gently close your eyes.
  I'd like you now to follow the suggestions that I am going to give, and let your mind act 'as if ...' ... as if what I am saying is really happening.
  I'd like you to visualise, sense and act as if I'm tying a huge bunch of helium balloons to your right wrist, and the balloons are tugging your wrist upward. Pulling and jerking, allowing your arm to rise ... easily... up and up ....
  Now imagine that I'm putting a large, heavy bucket into your left hand. Curl your fingers around the handle of the bucket. Hold it firmly as I now begin to fill the bucket with water. As you can imagine the water filling the bucket, the bucket becomes heavier and heavier. More and more water, heavier and heavier ... The bucket is SO heavy now that your left arm begins to pull downwards. You can feel the pull in your muscles.

Your right hand can continue to rise as the helium balloons keep tugging at your right wrist – lighter and lighter, your arm going up, higher and higher, up and up ....

Your left arm is SO heavy now. Feel the weight of the full bucket in your left hand. Left arm going down and down, heavier and heavier – even further down now ....

Right wrist going up, up and up. Lighter and lighter. The more you try to hold it down the more rapidly it rises, higher and higher, up and up.

Give yourself permission to follow your imagination.

You left arm is becoming really tired now. Feel the strain and the pull on your muscles, from your forearm all the way up to your shoulder. Left arm going down, and down and down. The bucket is SO heavy, it is difficult to hold it up.

Your right wrist is light, the balloons continue to rise, lighter and lighter, up and up and up.

Now, please open your eyes and notice your arms.

This exercise is great for demonstrating how the body will follow the instructions that the mind gives it. In a group, some people will have one arm down by their side and the other one right up in the air; with others, their arms will have only moved the smallest amount. There may even be people whose arms have not moved at all. If the sceptical person in the room is also the one whose arms have remained in their original position, they can be encouraged to look at their partner's arms and see how open to suggestion they are, and remind them that, while some people are very open to suggestion, it is impossible to make someone do something that they do not want to do.

Although Erikson used his technique as a means of induction, in hypnobirth this script is used as a convincer. When a person sees for themselves how they, or their partner, are affected by simple suggestions, they begin to understand the importance of language. This is one of the first exercises that the couples do and, even without any experience, let alone practice, of hypnosis they see how readily they will follow the suggestions of the person they see as the expert.

The brain, or computer, also reacts to external influences before it has consciously noticed the cause. For example, a person notices that they are feeling cold and decides to close the window, but what happened before they realised that they were feeling chilly? At first their brain will have registered the temperature gradually beginning to drop and it made adjustments to their circulation, moving the blood supply away from the skin and the extremities to conserve heat in the core so that their organs continued to function. This, in turn, caused a physical reaction on the surface of the skin and, when the reaction was large enough, the conscious part of the mind noticed that they were feeling cold and they got up and closed the window.

Although we have always known that the body reacts to our thoughts, this is now supported by neuroscience. Award-winning, pioneering neuroscientist Richard J. Davidson states in his book, *The Emotional Life of your Brain* (Davidson and Begley, 2012), that 'Feelings and thoughts, which originate in the brain, literally get out of that grey matter and into the rest of the body.' He explains that 'modern neuroscience has shown that emotions do infuse not only the mind but also the body. Feeling anxious raises your blood pressure and makes your pulse race, and feeling content can strengthen your immune system'.

Davidson offers the following examples:

'Fingernails screeching across a blackboard. A stiletto stabbing your eyeball ... and the blade of a knife being drawn slowly across the bottom of your foot. Did any of those set your teeth on edge?' (Davidson and Begley, 2012).

Here are a few more:

- Fear – if you are afraid of spiders or snakes and you imagine one moving towards your foot, how does your body respond?
- If you think about, or someone describes, a delicious meal, it might make your mouth water.
- The smell of a delicious meal may even make your stomach rumble.
- Flirting or sexy thoughts can produce all sorts of physical reactions; this is often more noticeable in men!
- Stress or anxiety can cause flushing or blotching on the neck or chest.
- Going for a job interview or speaking in public may cause your heart to race, your palms to become sweaty and your blood pressure to rise.

Birth rehearsal

For many people, rehearsal is an important component when preparing for an event. When anticipating an important job interview, we may rehearse our interview answers. Many athletes use rehearsal, otherwise known as visualisation, to improve sports performance. A study by Roure *et al.* (1998) showed that six specific autonomic nervous system (ANS) responses, related to mental rehearsal, showed an improvement in sports performance.

Davidson also relates his 'favourite example of how "mere" thought can change the brain in fundamental ways'; he tells how a group of Harvard University scientists led by Alvaro Pascual-Leone devised an experiment where a group of volunteers practise a simple keyboard piece over and over again for a week. At the end of the week, using neuroimaging, they discovered that the motor cortex responsible for moving those fingers had expanded. This discovery was much as they had expected it to be. However, what was interesting was that they had asked half of the group of volunteers to simply imagine playing the same notes over and over again, and they found that the same region had expanded in the same way. Davidson commented, 'Thinking, and thinking alone, had increased the amount of space the motor cortex devoted to a specific function' (Davidson and Begley, 2012).

Women who are pregnant can perform birth rehearsal using visualisation alongside the breathing and other practical techniques. However, if a woman believes that labour will be painful, she is much more likely to feel anxious, which can lead her into the fear–tension–pain cycle. The opposite is also true. If a woman is calm, and confident in her ability to relax and follow her instincts, she is much more likely to have that experience. This is especially true when she has practised the techniques that hypnobirth teaches her, and she understands how her body, and baby, can work together. These powerful hypnosis techniques are often used by athletes and by students working to pass important exams, and for many other life skills. The beauty of these techniques is that they translate well from hypnobirth for use in all sorts of areas of life.

Critical faculty of the conscious mind

We do not have easy access to the unconscious part of the mind as, during the first 5 or 6 years of life, we gradually develop something called the critical faculty of the conscious mind (Elman, 1964). Until this develops, young children cannot distinguish reality from imagination, which is why they have no trouble believing in Father Christmas and the Tooth Fairy. It is only as they reach this age that they begin to ask questions like, 'How does Santa manage to deliver presents to everyone in the whole world on Christmas Eve?' or 'What happens if there isn't a chimney?' They have begun to develop the ability to reason, and use logic, and they now start to distinguish between imagination and reality, based on everything they have learned so far. The conscious mind sets up a filter system which only accepts external ideas and suggestions, based on our current internal belief system.

In order to make changes to beliefs and habits using hypnosis, the critical faculty of the conscious mind must be bypassed, which allows access to the unconscious mind and negative beliefs can be released and replaced with positive ones. This can be done with relaxation, good information and positive language. Sometimes it can feel like an impossible task but, with determination, and practice, it is possible; occasionally additional hypnotherapy may be needed to release strong fears or anxieties.

In order for a new skill to become a habit, it must be practised over and over again, just as when someone is learning to ride a bike or drive a car. To begin with, they had to think about what they were doing and concentrate, focusing their attention on the details. Then they practised, and practised, until it became a habit. They now no longer need to think about how to ride a bike or drive a car. This happens whenever someone learns something new. In the meantime they have to act 'as if'.

Acting 'as if'

When someone starts a new job or learns a new skill they have to practise it over and over again until they become an expert. For example: they have been given a new responsibility at work, which means that they have to learn a new skill. Perhaps, as a newly trained hypnobirth midwife, they are standing in front of the first class that they are teaching on their own. It is really important to create a feeling of confidence in the group, so even if they are not feeling very confident, they must act 'as if' they are. Every time they teach a class, and act as if they are confident, their confidence will grow until one day they realise that they are no longer acting 'as if', but they really are confident. The more consciously this is done, the more effective the results will be.

Many women find hypnobirth through their fear of giving birth. The internal conversation they replay over and over again can include thoughts about pain, fear and not coping. Hypnobirth techniques teach a woman to act 'as if'. She is encouraged to focus on normality using affirmations, post hypnotic suggestions and a change of language. With practice, and over time, she will believe that birth can be much more comfortable. She will move from acting 'as if' she believes birth can be a positive experience, to actually believing it is possible. This is the power of hypnobirth.

Bibliography

Cowan, N. (2005). *Working memory capacity*. Hove: Psychology Press.

Cowan, N. (2001). The magical number 4 in short-term memory: A reconsideration of mental storage capacity. *Behav Brain Sci*, 24, 87–185.

Davidson, R. and Begley, S. (2012). *The emotional life of your brain*. New York: Hudson Street Press.

Elman, D. (1964). *Hypnotherapy*. London: Westwood Publishing.

Erickson, M. (1985). *The wisdom of Milton H. Erickson: Hypnosis and hypnotherapy*. New York: Irvington Publishers.

Erickson, M. (1958). Naturalistic techniques of hypnosis. *American Journal of Clinical Hypnosis*, 1, 3–8.

Freud, S. (1915). *The unconscious* (standard edn), 14, 159–204.

Krasner, A. (1990). *The wizard within*. Irvine, California: American Board of Hypnotherapy Press.

Leeman, L., Fontaine, P., King, V., Klein, M. and Ratcliffe, S. (2003). The nature and management of labor pain: Part I. Nonpharmacologic pain relief. *American Family Physician*, 68(6), 1109–1113.

Millar, G. (1956). The magical number seven, plus or minus two: Some limits on our capacity for processing information. *Psychological Review*, 63, 81–97.

Roure, R., Collet, C., Deschaumes-Molinaro, C., Dittmar, A., Rada, H. and Delhomme, G. (1998). Autonomic nervous system responses correlate with mental rehearsal in volleyball training. *Eur J Appl Physiol and Occupational Physiology*, 78(2), 99–108.

6

THE EFFECT OF LANGUAGE

Can words affect behavioural change? Words can calm, reassure, unite, divide and incite hatred or loyalty. We may believe our words, and language, to be harmless, but a 2007 study (Alia-Klein *et al.*) revealed that the words 'No' and 'Yes' can influence emotional behaviour and are associated with opposite brain responses. The word 'No' produced slower response times and evoked a negative signal in the right lateral orbitofrontal cortex (OFC). The OFC is the part of the brain involved in cognitive processing, emotion and decision making. The 'Yes' word produced faster response times and evoked a positive signal in a contiguous region of the OFC. Sowell *et al.* (2003) describe how the acquisition of language, and the emotional meaning of words, parallel frontal brain development. Research tells us that the way in which we respond to words, and language, can produce a physical, and emotional, response in our bodies. Positive language makes us strong, and powerful: you only have to listen to someone talking about a topic that they are passionate about. They will use positive words and be filled with positive energy and enthusiasm; this is infectious and has a powerful impact on the recipient.

Negative language has the opposite effect. Consider how you feel when you listen to someone who talks negatively about themselves, their work or their personal life. It can leave you feeling down and drained of energy. Have you ever experienced 'the moaner' at work? The person who is dissatisfied, unhappy and de-motivated. The moaner will complain to anyone who will listen. Sadly there is a tendency for others to join in and before you know it there is a whole group of moaners. Negativity, as well as positivity, spreads.

This kind of negative language eventually turns into a self-fulfilling prophecy. Negative words affect the physiology, and emotions, setting limits on what we believe we can achieve.

Barbara Fredrickson, one of the founders of Positive Psychology, discovered that we need to generate at least three positive thoughts and feelings for each expression of negativity. If you express fewer than three, personal and business relationships are likely to fail. This can be true of situations surrounding birth. Imagine that a woman arrives in early labour. She has been offered a vaginal examination. She accepts. Her cervix is found to be soft, fully effaced, anterior and one centimetre dilated. When this information is relayed to the woman, she will focus on what she sees as *only* one centimetre and discard the positivity of the fully effaced, soft anterior cervix. Of course, if words like effaced and anterior have been used, she may not have a clue what has been said!

BOX 6.1 SARAH'S STORY

The midwife whom I had asked not to give me a membrane sweep appeared from the 'examination' with very bloody hands and laughed, saying she had done 'a little sweep' whilst down there .... It's amazing how someone's words can belittle your requests and your rights to your body. I had been researching all week and had firmly decided against a sweep, seeing it as a major intervention. I felt disappointed by her actions but her words made me feel even more powerless.

Labour ward language

Hunter, in her 2006 article, argues that technological interventions and medical terminology become symbols of power in the hospital setting and reinforce the control of the provider at the expense of the woman. A study exploring midwives and their working environment revealed that the labour ward, and particularly the routines such as the admission procedure, gave the midwives a sense of power and control (Hunt and Symonds, 1995). Conrad and Schneider (1980) describe medicalisation as three distinct levels:

- **Conceptual level** – medical vocabulary is used. This is true of midwifery, with the jargon, abbreviations and medical terminology.
- **Institutional level** – organisations (NHS) adopt a medical approach in a specialist area (maternity).
- **Interactional level** – doctors are directly involved with defining, and diagnosing, a problem as medical. This can include treating a 'social' problem with a medical form of treatment (childbirth). This can also apply to communicating using medical terminology.

Think about the language that is used on the labour ward. Jargon in any setting can make people feel disempowered, and if a birthing couple are already feeling anxious, medicalised language can increase this anxiety. Hypnobirth couples learn relaxation techniques and use specific words which empower and build confidence. It would be helpful for birth professionals to continue the use of empowering language. Introducing this language into the culture at work will help all birthing women to feel more comfortable and relaxed.

The language used by birth professionals can be both confusing and a little overwhelming. Just reflect for a moment on the environment of obstetrics, and the language of that world. The journey of the baby through the pelvis is known as the 'mechanism of labour'. The implication is the body being a machine, with no connection to the mind, and emotions, of the woman. 'Active management' can be used to describe any stage of labour. The management is always by the institution, not the woman. This is illustrated by Hunter (2006), who uses an example of an article published in *Obstetrics and Gynaecology*: 'Induction of Labor in the Nineties: Conquering the Unfavourable Cervix'. The woman's body is often described in terms of parts. We talk about the cervix as if it has no connection to any other part of her body. Post-vaginal examination we often relay the information as 'you're five centimetres'. This implies that the cervix has taken over the woman. She is now five centimetres. The rest of her body is irrelevant. She is a walking cervix.

The word 'failure' seems to make an appearance a lot, with a 'failed induction', 'failure to progress', and a 'trial of scar'. The baby may become the focus of blame for some. We discuss babies being in the 'wrong' position if they deviate from the holy grail of LOA (left occiput anterior). We hear babies being described as 'naughty', 'lazy' and just not wanting to come out. There is a lack of recognition for the baby being the expert in the process.

BOX 6.2 MORE FROM SARAH

In labour I was transferred to hospital from a planned home birth due to high blood pressure. Once forced onto my back and strapped up to a cannula/drip, constant foetal monitoring, etc. (none were explained, just done to me), I was told repeatedly that 'baby is in a very tricky position and you will find it very hard to get this baby out', whilst other staff said 'you're progressing fine, baby has lots of hair!' Then another would say, 'this baby is in a very tricky position, you really will struggle to get baby out'. The negative attitude, after 9 months of reading and using positive hypnobirthing language, was disheartening and frustrating, made me feel that somehow baby and I had got it wrong. One positive midwife looked at me and said, 'this baby will come sooner than you think', but every time they examined me the sentence I got was, 'you are only 6cm', 'only 7cm', etc. My faith in myself and my body disappeared with every intervention and beep from the machinery, and the midwives rolling their eyes every time I tried to get onto all fours or lie on my side.

Language as control

It seems to be seen as a loss of power, control and status if we adjust the language to be inclusive. As a health professional you will be used to communicating with your colleagues using obstetric language. The hypnobirth philosophy requires the use of supportive, parent-friendly language. This can take practice and can be a challenge. Begin by listening to the language used when you are next at work. Start with the word 'delivered'.

Do you write it on the board? Could you change it to 'Birthed'?

How many times do you hear a midwife say, 'I've delivered'? This devalues the work of the woman. She did the hard work, not the midwife.

Do we identify women by characteristics other than their name?

- 'Room 2 needs an epidural.'
- 'The little primip in room 1 is contracting well.'
- 'The NCT woman wants a waterbirth.'
- 'The hypnobirther in room 6 doesn't want a VE.'
- 'The VBAC.'

The careless throwaway comment can be the most devastating of all. Here are some examples.

One hypnobirth couple experienced a caesarean birth with both of their boys. She came for hypnobirth with the second pregnancy as she had been so disappointed with her first experience. Although she subsequently had a second caesarean birth, she felt that her confidence in herself was much higher, and she and her birth partner had been involved in the decision-making process. The only moment where she felt let down was when she was sitting on her own with her new baby, staring into his eyes and feeling euphoric, and a midwife came in and said, 'Oh, you're the failed VBAC', and then left.

Another couple who were having their first baby and had practised the hypno-birth techniques over and over went into spontaneous labour. They drove to hospital when they were ready and gave birth in the early morning to a beautiful boy, in the birthing pool. The labour had lasted three-and-a-half hours and could be described as the perfect, normal birth. Later that day, having spent the time in a wonderful, oxytocin-filled bubble of delight, a newborn-hearing-screener arrived to check baby's hearing. She used her equipment and said that she couldn't get a reading, and left. Their bubble burst, the couple now thought that their baby was deaf, and the mother spent the rest of that day and all that night in tears.

No one had thought to explain to the couple that a negative test at this stage was quite normal.

The following day, another screener came to repeat the test, which showed that their baby's hearing was fine. The father was understandably furious at this careless, and unnecessary, lack of communication.

I had a call from a friend one day whose younger sister was pregnant; he was very upset and told me that the scan had shown that her baby was deformed. He began to tell me what had happened, but things didn't quite add up. He explained that she was a young, single mum, and her own mother wasn't able to make the appointment, so she had gone on her own. There was a trainee sonographer per-forming the ultrasound, who turned to her mentor and said, 'I can only see one arm and one leg'. Because they were engrossed in the images on the screen, neither of them saw the young woman go pale. When they had finished the scan, they sent her on her way without further comment. Now this scenario seemed unlikely, so I suggested that he talk to his sister, and mother, and that they contact the hospital for clarification. It turned out that the student could only see one arm and one leg because of the position of the baby, not because they weren't there. But because they were not paying enough attention, either to the pregnant woman, or to the language that they were using, they caused unnecessary distress to what should have been a moment of delight.

One woman was describing events that took place during her hypnobirth. Labour was induced, and the surges had slowed at 6cm. The midwife had discussed an oxytocin drip, and the hypnobirther had agreed that it was the best course of action. The midwife asked if she could 'put the drip up', but the woman was a little hesitant. She described not feeling ready. There were several more conversations like this over the next hour, with the woman in labour bracing herself for the drip to 'go up', and the midwife aiming for consent. She eventually agreed, and was surprised to find a cannula was needed in the back of her hand. Her expectation of 'putting the drip up' was that it was going up her vagina. This she did not feel ready for.

It is easy to think, 'I would never do that', but these are not isolated situations that have been described. As we all know, pregnant women can be incredibly sensitive, especially with regard to the safety of their babies, and sometimes what is said is not interpreted in the way that it was meant. We all have to take responsibility for our language and ensure that explanations are given carefully in everyday language that she will understand.

The language of midwives

Words and Phrases I've Heard Midwives Say That Need SCRAPPING. If you are a midwife and you use any of them … please consider other options:

- 'MY "ladies".'
- 'You might 'be ALLOWED' to have a home birth'… insert anything in for home birth. The language of permission is missing the point.
- 'I just catch babies'! Most midwives offer support based on reflected upon experience.
- 'If you don't push better than this I'm going to get the doctors'.
- Stop any references to 'stages' of 'labour' that suggests that they actually exist! Remember, we MADE them UP! Useful guide? Maybe? Maybe not.
- 'Pethidine will work well for you.'
- 'You must get on the bed for me to examine you.' 'If we put your legs into lithotomy you will be able to push better.'
- 'If you think this is painful [a comment on so-called latent phase of labour], just wait until "labour" starts.'
- With fingers in the woman's vagina: 'RELAX!'

- 'Just pop on the bed, I'm going to examine you "down there".'
- 'Chin on your chest, hold your breath and with the next contraction … PUUUUUUSH!'

Mark Harris (2015)

Hypnobirth language

Thoughts are the means by which we shape our experiences. We know that the mind reacts to language with emotion. The hypnobirth philosophy aims to use language that describes what is happening during the birthing experience in a gentler, non-medical manner.

We want to use words that evoke an emotion of feeling good, rather than fear and lack of understanding. Our words reinforce the belief that birth is a natural, normal life event (see table 6.1 for a comparison of medicalised and hypnobirth language).

We know from the definitions that hypnosis is a state of relaxation, and concentrated awareness, that is accompanied by an increased susceptibility to suggestion. It is important to remember, when the mind is relaxed and in this heightened state of suggestibility, to keep the suggestions positive. When a person has been in a state of hypnosis, even though they have emerged into a fully conscious state, they will still remain receptive to ideas, and suggestions, for 10 minutes or so. It is vital that you keep your couples' attention and continue to reinforce your positive messages during this time. When someone has been in a deep state of relaxation you can see that it takes a few minutes for them to really gather themselves together. Negative input at this stage can counteract the work that you have just been doing. This can happen after a relaxation session, a hypnobirth class and, most importantly, during labour.

TABLE 6.1 Hypnobirth language

Medicalised language	Hypnobirth language
Contraction	Surge
Pain	Sensation
Delivery	Birth
Pushing	Birth nudging
Effacing/dilating	Thinning/opening
Patients	Clients
Braxton Hicks	Pre-labour warm ups
Fully dilated	Fully open
Sweep	Cervical massage
Primips/Multips	1st-/2nd-time mums
Transition	Near completion
Trial of scar/VBAC	Birth after caesarean
C-Sections	Caesarean birth
Home confinement	Home birth
ARM	Membrane release

I remember one occasion when I was packing up after holding a class in the Midwifery Led Unit (MLU) of the local hospital. After the couples had left, one of the midwives came in with a couple who had arrived to take a tour of the unit. Unfortunately it was full, but the midwife asked if I could spare them a few minutes, as it was possible that one of the rooms might become available quite soon. I invited the couple in for a chat, and it was soon apparent that they were both rather anxious about the birth. I explained a little bit about hypnobirth, did a short relaxation with them and taught them a simple breathing technique. In all we spent about 40 minutes, during which time I had offered them a lot of suggestions to relieve their anxiety and to sow the seed that she could be calm, confident and relaxed, which could lead to a much more comfortable experience.

They were both considerably more relaxed as we walked back to the reception area. There was a member of staff sitting behind the desk who explained that the rooms were all still busy. She then asked if they had enjoyed their brief session with me, they were all smiles, and said that they had and that it had been really interesting. I was delighted to have been able to sow a few small, and positive, seeds that I hoped would take root and grow. Unfortunately, the member of staff then said, 'That's great; of course it won't make any difference to your pain'. Their faces fell, the anxiety was back in full and it was apparent that in one short sentence she had undone everything we had achieved in the last 40 minutes. Please be aware that it can be easy to 'derail' a labouring woman, which is why hypnobirth puts so much emphasis on the language used, not only in class, but especially during labour and birth.

Although I couldn't change the experience for that couple, it prompted me to talk to the head of the MLU and to arrange an introductory session for the midwives and other staff in the unit. It also cemented my belief in the importance of sharing these techniques with as many birth professionals as possible: not only the ones who will teach the classes, but also those who attend women during pregnancy, and birth, so that we can transform birth together, and enable women, their birth partners and, of course, their babies to have the very best experience, no matter what happens.

One of the reasons why mothers, and their birth partners, want to come to an antenatal class is because they feel anxious, which might simply be due to lack of knowledge. It is normal to fear the unknown. For some, though, it will be because something else has made them anxious or afraid. This could be a past experience, listening to negative birth stories and, of course, seeing birth portrayed negatively by the media. It is interesting that, as soon as a couple becomes pregnant, it seems that everyone wants to share their birth stories, no matter how negative their experience may have been. Sometimes the more negative the story, the more gleefully it is told. It can be that telling stories where we have overcome adversity can make us feel brave and will often induce sympathy in our audience. This is known as secondary gain.

I once had a client who came to see me because throughout her life she had regularly been in accidents that were a result of her own clumsiness. It had started when she was little; she always remembered being clumsy, her mother often called her clumsy, and eventually whenever she bumped into something she would tell herself that she was clumsy, and so the belief was formed. One day, whilst still a child, she had an accident and broke her leg. She was in a cast, and fairly immobile for several weeks, during which time her mother paid her lots of attention and was nicer to her than usual, which made her feel very special. Over the years a pattern developed that meant that, whenever she had a fairly serious accident, people would rally round her, and look after her, reminding her of that feeling when she had felt very special.

By the time she came to me she had experienced a series of quite serious accidents, and her husband and their daughter had always taken special care of her. However, this belief was now beginning to conflict with a strong desire to be well and to look after her husband and daughter. She began to feel resentful of, and a little guilty about, these accidents, resulting in her coming to me to see if I could help her be less clumsy. It took a little while to unravel her story; she thought it was a matter of balance and paying better attention. When we began to discuss the idea that secondary gain might be part of the problem, she was furious. My first thought was that she was furious with me for suggesting such a thing – it can be difficult to hear. But she wasn't; she was livid that she had spent so much of her life injured, in the hope that she might feel special and cared for. She made an instant decision to change and went home to tell her husband and daughter, who both adored her, that when she hurt herself they were to ignore her as much as possible in order to help her learn that the consequence of clumsiness was just pain and that there was no longer any secondary gain. They agreed, although they found it quite hard. She continued to work with me, and as we gradually changed this belief, she became less and less clumsy. We created new affirmations that reinforced her new belief and, in time, her old clumsy habits were a distant memory and she had a wonderful loving family who looked after each other in good health.

So now we have some understanding of why people want to share their traumatic stories. Unfortunately, the effect that these stories have on a newly pregnant woman can range from mild anxiety to utter devastation. It is not usually enough for a single negative story to cause utter devastation, but when it is compounded by other negative reinforcement it can lead to tokophobia. Considering all the negative input that a young woman may have received, it is perhaps not surprising that she would feel such a deep level of anxiety and fear. Her fear is not so much irrational, as an unbalanced view of pregnancy and birth.

There have been several women who have been described as tokophobic and referred for hypnosis by their community midwife with symptoms of severe anxiety, including uncontrolled crying, shaking and sweating at the thought of giving birth. On more than one occasion the original trigger was seeing a graphic video of birth, in their teens, during a class at school. Their memory of the class was that pregnancy and birth would be their 'punishment' if they engaged in sexual activity. The overall message of abstinence was being delivered in an effort to prevent teenage pregnancy but, for some, the message was delivered too powerfully.

There are women who have worked in high-risk obstetric units, and special care baby units, where all they have seen is the very high-risk end of the pregnancy, labour and birth spectrum. As a result, their vision became skewed because they had seen very little, or no, normal labour and birth. It is not surprising that they were so fearful. What we experience affects our imagination of our future.

However, the biggest influence, by far, in creating anxiety and fear in pregnancy is the media portraying dramatised images of birth, and of course the reality TV birth programmes. In 2013 Kathrin Stoll and Wendy Hall conducted a study of 2,676 young women who had not given birth but planned to do so in the future that explored predictors of childbirth fear. It was found that those who were influenced by the media were one-and-a-half times more likely to report a fear of childbirth. It was also found that fear of childbirth was reduced with a woman's confidence in her knowledge of pregnancy, labour and birth.

Until relatively recently, birth was the domain of the women in the extended family as well as the community midwives and occasionally the family doctor. Young women, and girls, would experience birth long before they had children of their own. They would have seen or heard about a wide variety of home births and would have had a much more realistic view of the process.

If the emotion that we experience when we first learn about something is very strong, it will be stored in our unconscious mind and will reveal itself whenever we think of, or find ourselves in, a similar situation. So the young school girl adversely affected by a graphic video of birth will recreate that feeling each time she thinks about having a baby. This strengthens the feelings of fear, revulsion or whatever she felt, until the thought of pregnancy, and childbirth, is terrifying. This is how limiting beliefs are formed. Every negative birth story she hears, or overly dramatised traumatic TV birth that she sees, will reinforce this limiting belief. However, even though she was troubled by that first experience, if her subsequent exposure to birth had been positive, she would eventually be able to release the negative feelings. With hypnobirth she will be immersed in positive language, DVDs and birth stories as well as receiving hypnosis to release the fear and excellent antenatal education. With plenty of practice and the support of her confident birth partner, her beliefs will change, and she can achieve a positive birth experience, which will further reinforce her new positive beliefs.

The power of suggestion

Large corporations are well aware of the power of language, and suggestion, and they spend billions every year on advertising their products to us. Just think about it for a moment: while watching the television, every 15 minutes or so we are told over and over again by people we might admire, or even aspire to be, that we need this product or that service. If it didn't work, these huge organisations wouldn't spend all those billions every year!

Some of the most powerful suggestions that influence us are the stories that we tell ourselves:

- 'I'm hopeless at remembering names.'
- 'I never sleep well, unless I'm at home in my own bed.'
- 'I can't do maths.'
- 'I always lose my car keys.'
- 'I can't find my phone.'
- 'I'm not good enough.'

I expect you can think of all sorts of stories that you tell yourself. Just like habits, every time we repeat the story, we reinforce it, and the mind finds ways to make it come true.

Learning styles

There are three learning styles, and most people have a dominant style. If you listen to the words that are used you will notice which style individuals learn from most effectively. The three styles are visual, auditory and kinaesthetic.

Visual learners will use language that relates to vision – do you *see* what I mean, how does that *look* to you? They respond best to suggestions like, *picture* yourself; you may *see* a shell or a pebble.

Auditory learners will use language that relates to hearing – how does that *sound*? This kind of learner will respond to *listening* suggestions: *hear* the sound of water; *listen* to the birds singing.

Kinaesthetic learners respond to touch and texture – how does that *feel*? *Feel* the warm sand; *brush* your hand across the *waxy* leaves.

Scripts need to have a mixture of these learning styles, so that the group can get the most out of them. Scripts also use neutral words, like imagine, notice and sense – *imagine*, *notice* or have a *sense* of the sand under your feet: a visual person might see it, an auditory person might hear it crunch and a kinaesthetic person would feel the texture.

Even though one style may be dominant, people use all styles to a degree, and by mixing the styles as you talk to couples, they will have the best opportunity to learn.

Positive words

Why do we change our words for hypnobirth?

Positive words and language make us strong, and powerful; you only have to listen to someone talking about a topic that they are passionate about. They will use positive words and be filled with positive energy and enthusiasm; this is infectious and has a powerful impact on the recipient.

Negative language has the opposite effect. Consider how you feel when you listen to someone who talks negatively about themselves, their work or their personal life. It can leave you feeling down and drained of energy.

Language is such an important part of hypnobirth; it underpins every aspect: the scripts, the affirmations and the words that are used during the classes and with the couples that you work with during their labour and birth.

Consider the following sentences:

- 'When I examined you, you were **only** 4cm dilated.'
- 'I'm **just** a stay-at-home mum.'
- 'I'm **still** in the same job.'

It is the words **only**, **just** and **still** that will have an effect on the recipient. Small words can change the entire feel of a conversation.

Remember to think about the language that you use on the labour ward. Introducing positive language into the culture at work will help all birthing women to feel more comfortable and relaxed.

Positive statements and affirmations

The positive statements and affirmations that are used in hypnobirth are a very powerful way of allowing your clients to continually self-motivate when they are on their own. Of course, you may help the mother to create her own statements. They must be personal, positive, precise, plausible and written in the present, and they must be practised.

Here are a few examples:

- With every out breath I can double my relaxation.
- As I focus on my breathing my body responds with complete relaxation.
- Each day I grow more and more confident that my birth will be calm and comfortable.
- Every time I practise my relaxation it will be easier, quicker and deeper.
- I feel my body softening, relaxing and releasing with every surge.

Affirmations can be used by your clients as positive mantras and repeated as often as suits them to help maintain a positive and confident mindset; this helps them to act 'as if' until it becomes a new belief.

Avoid negative suggestions. The brain does not do negatives. If I say to you, 'Don't think of a pink elephant', what's the first thing that comes into your mind?

Recently I was staying in a hotel and was chatting with one of the members of staff, a very friendly young woman, called Aggie. I asked Aggie whether she was working the following day; she pulled a bit of a face and said that she was on the early shift, which meant that she would have to get up at 6.30am. Now Aggie was very energetic and efficient, but didn't really like early mornings and never slept very well the night before. When I asked her why, she told me that she worried that she wouldn't wake up on time. So, the evening before, the thoughts going through her head were, 'I won't wake up, I'm going to be late. What if I don't hear the alarm? I'll get into trouble.' These thoughts would whir around her head until eventually she would fall asleep only to wake a few hours later to repeat these same thoughts. This would typically happen two or three more times before she had to get up, feeling tired and lethargic. I suggested that she might like to try something different. Instead of her usual thoughts, she should simply say, 'I will wake at 6.30, I will wake at 6.30, I will wake at 6.30' and, if she awoke in the night, to repeat it again as she quickly fell asleep.

The next morning I went down to breakfast and was greeted by a grinning Aggie, who told me that she had done as I suggested and had had the best night's sleep she'd had in ages, and had woken up at 6.30am on the dot feeling fantastic! She had told all the other members of staff on duty, who wanted to know if I had any other tips for tiredness and insomnia! Incidentally I also woke at 6.30am because I had neglected to change the thought in my own mind after explaining the process to Aggie – I think that comes under the heading of 'be careful what you wish for'.

Here's one to try at home. As your partner leaves the house, you might say, 'Don't forget the milk', in which case they are very likely to forget the milk. If you say, 'Remember the milk when you go out', they are much more likely to do so. In an affirmation, instead of 'I will not feel any pain', the affirmation should be 'I will feel comfortable and relaxed', which will allow the body to follow the mind's suggestion.

As you go about your work, or your everyday life tasks, begin to notice the language of others. Be mindful of your own language and just notice the power of your words. You have the ability to change a birth with your words. Use it wisely.

References

Alia-Klein, N., Goldstein, R. Z. and Tomasi, D. (2007). What is in a word? No versus yes differentially engage the lateral orbitofrontal cortex. *Emotion* (Washington, DC), 649–659.

Conrad, P. and Schneider, J. (1980). *Deviance and medicalisation: From badness to sickness.* (1st edn). St Louis, Missouri: Mosley.

Harris, M. (2015, August 5th). Midwives: 17 words and phrases to stop using .... Please!, Birthing for Blokes: http://birthingawareness.com/?s=midwives+language. Retrieved July 3rd 2015.

Hunt, S. and Symonds, A. (1995). In O. Povey-Edmondson (ed.), *The social meaning of midwifery*. Houndmills: Macmillan Press.

Hunter, L. (2006). Women give birth and pizzas are delivered: Language and Western childbirth paradigms. *Journal of Midwifery and Women's Health*, 119–124.

Sowell, E. R., Peterson, B. S., Thompson, P. M., Welcome, S. E., Henkenius, A. L. and Toga, A. W. (2003). Mapping cortical change across the human life span. *Natural Neuroscience*, 309–315.

Stoll, K. and Hall, W. (2013). Vicarious birth experiences and childbirth fear: Does it matter how young Canadian women learn about birth? *The Journal of Perinatal Education – Advancing Normal Birth*, 22(4), 226–233.

7

RELATIONSHIPS

The ways in which humans grow and change in the womb, and in the days, weeks and months after they are born, are influenced by genetic, environmental, emotional and cognitive factors. Early intervention, in the form of antenatal education, directly affects a child's immediate and long-term health, emotional development, socialisation, relationships and educational achievements (Barlow *et al.*, 2009).

There is good evidence that antenatal education can help manage and reduce maternal anxiety and depression during pregnancy. However, little has been written on men's perception of childbirth and the changing relationships in pregnancy. Outcomes of antenatal education have historically focused on maternal benefits. Fathers, in one study, reported antenatal classes to be unhelpful, and in some cases they increased their fears (Hanson *et al.*, 2009).

Hypnobirth encourages a couple to practise scripts, relaxation and deepening techniques. Each class includes practice and work to do at home. We know that repetition is the key to success for hypnobirthing couples, and teachers actively encourage home practice.

Kerry says:

> Me and my husband very much enjoyed practising the hypnobirthing techniques. It was a time of calm and relaxation that we both looked forward to every day, and I loved the fact that it felt we were working as a team towards a common goal. This feeling continued through the labour itself – with my husband able to play a very active role in the entire process. The techniques he had learnt meant that he was a very reassuring and comforting presence throughout my birth experience.
>
> Our (very calm and placid) baby is now 5 months old, but we got so much out of practising the techniques that we are continuing to do some of the

practices now and again, in order to regain that special 'couple' time, and just take a few minutes out of the busy day to fully relax.

Melissa and David say:

> My partner and I did the hypnobirthing classes. We are first-time parents and found that not only did the classes bring us closer; it also made him feel part of the pregnancy.
>
> He had been finding it difficult not knowing how to help me, as I had a difficult start to the pregnancy. We found the classes brought us closer and also calmed us both down so we know we can handle the birth and the baby. We are yet to have our baby but we practise daily and know we are ready for the Journey.

A descriptive study in Finland included 137 fathers. All the men had attended at the birth of their child, and the study asked about the experience of childbirth and how the fathers felt. The greatest concern was 'how their partner would cope during birth'. This was closely followed by 'feelings of helplessness', 'concern for the well-being of the baby', and 'fears that their partner might die' (Vehvilainen-Julkunen and Liukkonen, 1998).

BOX 7.1 CLAIRE AND ANDY'S STORY

At a time when I was so scared and frightened, hypnobirthing worked wonders. It calmed me and helped me to focus, but, as a completely unexpected bonus, it was amazing for our relationship. It made us stronger and helped myself and my husband to be a team. He had to know what I wanted inside out. He had to be able to speak for me when I was at my most vulnerable. He was responsible for communicating for me and our baby and we relied on him to be our voice. My job was to birth our baby; his was to be the facilitator between us and the hospital staff, look after us and to instinctively respond for us. Initially, we feared that he would not even be able to attend the birth, such is his deep paralyzing fear of hospitals! I could not be more proud of him, as he fully embraced hypnobirthing and was my absolute rock. Hypnobirthing works for men too!

A total of 20 men took part in a 2007 Swedish study examining men's fear surrounding childbirth. When men fear birth, it can manifest as catastrophic thoughts, and their main concern was the health and life of their partner and child. Despite the fear, all of the men had attended the birth and described why, in terms of 'responsibility', 'involvement' and 'obligation'. Interestingly most of the men had not discussed their fears with their partner before birth (Eriksson et al., 2007). Pregnancy is a complex time, with most couples facing many changes physically, emotionally and psychologically. Antenatal education cannot provide enough time to fully explore the changing relationships, nor was it designed to do so. However, there are windows of opportunity to encourage reflection and communication. Some hypnobirth courses include a session on pre-birth bonding. This can be instinctive to most parents, but some struggle to identify ways of connecting with their unborn. As advances in neuroscience have better increased our understanding of the links between early brain development and later life outcomes, the more opportunities that parents have to experience this, the better. Fear release is an integral aspect in hypnobirth. The course encourages parents to write a list of fears surrounding birth, separately, and then to compare lists. Often couples can be surprised by the other's anxieties. There is an opportunity to share the fears in class and work with a fear release script. This session can often end with tears, and many women have commented on how cathartic it can feel.

Parents participating in one study reported surprise at the changes in the relationship with their partner. The men reported feeling very involved with their partners' pregnancy but excluded from antenatal appointments, antenatal classes and by the literature that was available (Deave *et al.*, 2008). One point of interest is that some men felt excluded by not being given contact details for midwives, hospitals, health visitors. They felt the emphasis was focused on the woman. When an invitation is sent for antenatal classes, it is often addressed to the woman. Literature and information is aimed at the pregnant woman. As health professionals, it can be all too easy to reduce the woman to a bed number, and when we do remember her name, we often do not include the birth partner. We can blame time constraints, but by excluding the partner we deny the existence of the family.

BOX 7.2 MORE FROM CLAIRE AND ANDY

Through weeks and weeks (I was 18 days overdue so we had more time than most!), we gradually became the strongest team. We spent every night practising scripts, massage techniques and listening to the hypnobirth affirmation and relaxation CD. This time that we spent together was invaluable to us as a couple. We didn't realise it at the time, but it made us have quality time together before the birth that we probably would never have had. I will always cherish that time dearly. I was so confident that we were on the same page, that he also wrote my birth plan for me. It brought us so close together and completely allayed our fears.

A few weeks after I found out I was pregnant, the reality of the birth started to creep in. I was panic stricken, tearful and felt quite alone. Hypnobirthing brought us from that to a place where I completely embraced the notion of birthing, looked forward to it and had actually planned on a home birth! I felt so close to my husband as we had come through that journey together and we became far stronger because of it. That in itself was worth its weight in gold. We have since gone on to have another child using hypnobirthing and he was right by my side again. Absolutely amazing.

Historically it has been paid-for antenatal education such as National Childbirth Trust classes that have encouraged small groups, class interaction and post-natal support. More recently we have seen NHS classes adopting this model, and hypnobirth classes can facilitate the social support that couples will require postnatally.

> Social support acts as a buffer that helps an individual cope better with stressful situations. The transition to parenthood is unquestionably such a time. The quality of social support available to parents is therefore an important factor in their adjustment to their new role.
>
> *(Montigny et al., 2006)*

Although couples arrive at hypnobirth prepared to learn labour skills, they leave having completed a journey with others, laughing, sharing and comparing. These relationships often last years and provide superb support in early parenthood. There are exceptions, and these can depend on the group size. Many private hypnobirth practitioners teach one-to-one sessions. In terms of time and convenience, this is a popular option. However, the lack of shared learning and support network can be a disadvantage. There are hypnobirth classes taught that far exceed the standard 'ideal group' number. Larger classes enable sub-group work; however, anything larger than eight couples results in a lecture, rather than an interactive session. Six couples is a reasonable size for a participative group and allows subdivision by twos. By the very nature of the topic, antenatal classes result in discussion around some intimate body parts that many couples may not be prepared for. Birth cannot be discussed without talking about vaginas, bodily functions and sometimes sex. The group will need to feel comfortable and relaxed enough to be able to ask questions. One hypnobirth course was attended by 16 couples. A group with 32 people in it is an audience; no one remembers anyone's name and interaction is limited. The relationship that the teacher builds within the first session is crucial. She is building trust and gaining confidence. The couples will then feel confident enough to relax, ask questions and gain from the group what they need.

BOX 7.3 NICOLA AND DANIEL'S STORY

Due to my medical conditions I was considered medium risk and under the care of the consultants. After attending hypnobirthing classes Daniel and I both had a much more positive outlook on labour. We knew that there may be complications and we might need to give birth in an obstetrics room. However, we were both determined that no matter what happened we would be able to use the hypnobirthing techniques we had learnt.

When we watched the hypnobirthing video Daniel and I both felt emotional and realised just how beautiful birth could be.

Hypnobirthing definitely brought us much closer through the pregnancy. Daniel felt that he could share the experience with me. Our baby loved the deep breathing techniques and would start dancing around. Because my placenta was anterior, and after birth we found out larger than average, Daniel couldn't always feel her move when I could. However, when we practised breathing with the three-hand touch, Daniel could feel her wriggling around even when I couldn't. It brought him closer to our baby as well as to me. I loved seeing his face light up when he could feel her move.

My labour lasted 68 hours, during which we wanted to create a memorable birth story that we would never forget, rather than just focusing on the last few hours in hospital. Hypnobirthing changed our mindset from simply waiting to go to hospital to a more positive and active latent phase of labour that we could both enjoy. Once labour began we continued the walks we had enjoyed throughout pregnancy.

On the second day of labour we went for a wonderful and very slow, fun 5-hour walk down by the Colne River, through to the castle park, watched *Frozen* on the big screen, had an ice cream, cup of tea, fed a squirrel and walked back.

I know that having a partner that is actively involved in the hypnobirthing makes a big difference. For each surge Daniel wasn't with me, they felt more intense and more difficult to manage. Even when my eyes were closed, knowing he was there made it easier. He became my rock standing by my side and holding my hand through each surge till Millie was in the world.

Can the success of hypnobirth be influenced by relationships? Yes undoubtedly. The couple attending the course need to work together antenatally, practising the techniques, discussing worries and fears, and adapting to their ever-changing relationship. Hypnobirth can encourage and facilitate this communication.

The hypnobirthing couple relationship

A birth partner can make or break a birth. Many midwives know this. How many times do we send an unhelpful partner out for a walk, a sandwich, a cigarette, only to have a baby whilst they are gone? Michel Odent is a famous supporter of removing unhelpful men from the birthing room. He suggests that women may verbalise their need for partner support, but their non-verbal language, their body language, often tells a different story. If birth proves to be primal, vocal, sweaty and loud, does the presence of an unprepared partner hinder the process?

It is essential that the birth supporter gets on board with hypnobirth if that is the kind of birth the woman wants. Some couples bring a third supporter to classes, a mum, doula, sister, or friend. They will all be crucial in maintaining the birth room space and should be involved with the practice. The couple with unresolved issues, including relationship problems, previous birth experience trauma or general lack of support will not do as well as those who have worked through these issues.

BOX 7.4 DANIELLE AND PAUL'S STORY

We began our hypnobirthing journey at about 25 weeks of pregnancy. Up to this point, whilst loving each other, there had been frustrations between my husband and me. I felt he was unsympathetic to the terror I felt at the prospect of the gory birth I 'knew' I was destined for. He, in turn, admitted a total lack of understanding and was taking a lead from my terror, a situation that was causing growing angst between us as the weeks rolled by.

We had our first hypno class with a wonderful midwife. We were under this cloud and sceptical about what it could really do to help, if anything. Hypnobirthing not only taught us the techniques but, more importantly, it brought us closer together. It showed my husband how to be helpful and supportive, and removed the fear from my mind, so I could see him there, willing to do whatever he could to help me, and that I was absolutely not in it alone. We learnt it was ok to laugh, ask questions and relax together. I could give my worries to him and take control of our care but, most importantly, it empowered us both to understand that my husband could be my protector and a massive support in a situation where he believed himself to be irrelevant and powerless. Together we learned skills to manage this wonderful impending event of our first baby's arrival. Removing all the stigma of birth, anxiety became genuine excitement, clipped conversations between us became free flowing dialogues, tension became ease and even smiles, and laughter was once again a regular fixture between us when discussing the birth.

By the time our turn arrived, we were calm, practised in our roles, relaxed and ready for it. Evie's birth did not go the way we would have hoped, but it didn't matter, we were undeterred, focused and used our hypnobirthing skills that proved wonderful in keeping us calm, together and in control. We were elated to welcome our beautiful daughter safely, side by side and stronger than ever. Neither of us can wait to do it again.

Hypnobirth teacher–client relationship

The relationship between the hypnobirth facilitator and the class is an important one. The group need to feel confident in the ability of the teacher. They need to believe hypnobirth will work, to engage with the practice. The teacher must be comfortable and confident in her own skills, engage the group and know when to withdraw from the group. Responding to the needs of the group and evolving with the group is a skill. This is called matching and pacing in hypnosis terms, but is just as essential for group work. This is where we know that class size matters. She needs to be aware of every member of the group and their reaction to the topic. Often the subject matter is intimate, emotional or both. Confidentiality is made clear and should be set out initially as part of consolidating a safe environment. Another important aspect is managing expectation and giving couples a realistic picture of birth. Hypnobirth will focus on the normality of birth, but can rehearse different scenarios in order to consider which techniques might be most appropriate. Hypnobirth can be used for all births, and when birth moves in a different or difficult direction it is those women who really value the techniques.

There are three 'types' of hypnobirth teacher:

- the hypnobirthing mum. This is the woman who has experienced hypnobirth for her own labour and now wants to spread the word. She has no midwifery or hypnotherapist training;
- the hypnotherapist who wants to expand their practice to include birth;
- midwives.

The skills of a hypnobirth teacher can be varied; all are useful. Having experienced hypnobirth herself, the hypnobirthing mum will bring authenticity and real birth experience. The hypnotherapist is an expert in the field, and the midwife is ideally placed to teach hypnobirth.

Women will seek out the practitioner that best meets their needs. Some women prefer a course provided in their home by non-medical staff. They want to escape the medical model and do not find attending classes in a hospital environment relaxing. Many others find NHS branding reassuring and seek courses taught by midwives in hospitals. The relationship between teacher and client can be a powerful one. We have seen couples consult with the hypnobirth teacher whilst in labour rather than the midwife. This highlights the depth of trust that the relationship can yield and therefore the importance of the right information during classes.

There can be a sense of setting couples a 'them' and 'us' divide. Hypnobirth has historically been seen as 'alternative' and provided by private practitioners. The birth philosophy can be misaligned with the NHS medical model. Couples have arrived ready for confrontation, for the 'fight' to achieve their normality. They may be surprised to learn that midwives want the kind of birth that they want. Bringing hypnobirth into the NHS has diluted much of the 'fight'. Hypnobirth has not changed, and the philosophy is one that midwives have always strived to achieve.

The success of hypnobirth is multifaceted, and there are many variables that can influence the birth outcome other than hypnosis. Couples who have researched hypnobirth and invested time and often a lot of money in a course may be more likely to report success. The Mongan method states that '50% of hypnosis happens before the client attends classes', and this is supported by our experience. Women and partners who are motivated will benefit the most. When hypnobirth is offered free within the NHS there are many couples who 'just try it'. Removing the cost can devalue the course, and we have found more women signing up and not turning up, or attending without any understanding of the work required. However, these are few, and the majority are prepared to work at their skills. Offering hypnobirth free within the NHS promotes equity, choice and, most importantly, normality.

BOX 7.5 JAMES AND LOUISE'S STORY

James about Louise

Many years ago, in the early stages of our relationship, Louise and I had a major row. I had asked her what her ambition in life was, and she had said it was to have a baby. I told her that this wasn't actually an ambition because any woman can have a baby. An ambition needed to be something difficult to achieve that you had to work hard for.

In retrospect, it isn't surprising that this did not go down well. But even before we started hypnobirthing, Louise's struggle with endometriosis had made me realise how naive I was to think that every woman can simply fall pregnant at will. More significantly, hypnobirthing taught me that preparing properly to birth a baby in the way that you want and that you believe is best for your baby is truly an inspiring and magical achievement. I couldn't have been prouder of Louise: from the way she planned and practised to the confidence and patience with which she approached breastfeeding afterwards. And I was honoured to have been a part of that whole process.

Hypnobirthing encouraged us to see birth precisely as a joint achievement. The classes and the practice brought us closer than we had ever been, such that when labour started we immediately drew together to put into practice what we had worked for so long on. I felt Louise's trust in me, which boosted my trust in myself, and enabled me to feel fully part of what was happening and to support her further. For a woman who rarely accepts support from anyone, this was a massive deal! In the weeks before birth, a friend we had invited to dinner tried to prepare me, based on his experience of his son being born, that unless I was medically trained I would feel like a spare part in the process. Hypnobirthing had prepared me that this was some fathers' experience, but it didn't have to be mine. It wasn't, and whilst I can't deny that Louise did all the hard work on the day, I feel immensely proud of our achievements. And, of course, of our amazing son Freddie, 8lb 11oz.

Louise about James

I have suffered endometriosis for around 10 years, during which time I have had four laparoscopy procedures, been through the menopause twice and had a marina coil. To say our journey for a baby was easy would be wrong, but it wasn't the hardest either. It put a certain amount of strain on our relationship, I don't think a man can ever truly understand a woman and her maternal instinct, but we constantly tried to remain strong and positive. As soon as I found out I was pregnant I knew I wanted to hypnobirth and I wanted that to be at home. I didn't want our baby to be born in a clinical environment and I also wanted a break from that myself. James wanted to support me in whatever I decided was best.

I'm not sure what we expected when starting hypnobirthing but I know it's changed our relationship forever. We learnt to be a team in a way I could never imagine. I have never been very good at being comforted or accepting help, even from my husband. It's something that's also proved tough for him to accept. Hypnobirthing encouraged me to let go and trust him, trust he can soothe and relax me, calm me when I needed him to and support me unconditionally.

We practised the mantras, light touch massage and rebozo work a lot! I'm glad we did. When I went into labour we understood each other's roles and calmly created our environment, one of peace and love, to meet our son. My labour wasn't easy, my surges were very intense. I lost my breathing and focus sometimes but James was there, right by my side all the time. A gentle shoulder anchor would focus me, affirmations playing on the laptop reminding me why we're doing this, positive talks to confirm that this is achievable and we were going to meet our son.

Freddie was born at 21.27. After the birth, and the days following, it was like I'd seen James for the first time. I fell in love with him all over again. I was in love with the man who had been on my team through labour and even more so with the man I'd watched transition into a father. If I have a tough day and think 'I can't do this', he reminds me I can, or that I am doing it; he tells me daily I'm doing a great job and I tell him. I knew I'd feel an overwhelming love for my son but I never knew what would also happen to my relationship.

People ask me about hypnobirthing and what it's about, I tell them it's a state of mind, it's about what you can do as a team.

References

Barlow, J., Coe, C., Redshaw, M. and Underdown, A. (2009). Birth and beyond: Stakeholder perceptions of current antenatal education provision in England. London: Department of Health. http://webarchive.nationalarchives.gov.uk/20130107105354/http://www.dh.gov.uk/prod_consum_dh/groups/dh_digitalassets/documents/digitalasset/dh_109831.pdf.

Deave, T., Johnson, D. and Ingram, J. (2008, July 28th). Transition to parenthood: The needs of parents in pregnancy and early parenthood. Biomedcentral: www.biomedcentral.com/1471-2393/8/30. Retrieved August 14th 2015.

Eriksson, C., Westman, G. and Hamberg, K. (2007). Content of childbirth-related fear in Swedish women and men – Analysis of an open-ended question. *Journal of Midwifery and Women's Health*, 112–118.

Hanson, S., Hunter, L. P., Bormann, G. and Sobo, E. (2009). Paternal fears of childbirth: A literature review. *The Journal of Perinatal Education*, 12–20.

Montigny, F., Lacharité, C. and Amyot, E. (2006). The transition to fatherhood: The role of formal and informal support structures during the post partum period. *Texto Contexto Enferm*, 601–609.

Vehvilainen-Julkunen, K. and Liukkonen, A. (1998). Fathers' experiences of childbirth. *Midwifery*, 10–17.

8

BREATHING TECHNIQUES FOR BIRTH

The hypnobirth course is made up of key components, and one of them is breathing techniques. Many midwives may remember relaxation taught as progressive muscle relaxation. This was first introduced by American physician Edmund Jacobson in the early 1920s. From the 1950s until the 1970s in antenatal classes across the country 'the breathing' was taught to mothers. This practice lost popularity during the last decade, but a 2006 American survey reported that 25 per cent of all women giving birth used relaxation techniques, with nearly 50 per cent using breathing techniques. The Lamaze technique is especially popular in the USA, with its roots in Russian psychoprophylaxis.

The relaxation response

Dr Herbert Benson coined the term the 'relaxation response' during the 1960s and 70s. His work studied the scientific benefits of relaxation on a wide range of stress-related disorders. Benson reveals that a state of deep rest changes the physical and emotional response to stress. When lecturing on the relaxation response, Benson (1975) uses physical movement to illustrate:

> You know how when you play an instrument and you become 'one' with that instrument and the time flits away? That is the relaxation response. You know the high you get from running? That is the relaxation response coming about by the repetitive motion of your footfall.

Labouring women when left undisturbed have reported feelings of euphoria, of 'being on another planet', of 'zoning out'. Breath control can assist them to achieve this relaxation response quickly.

It has been known for many years that slowing the breath is beneficial. A calm, relaxed breath is associated with a calm psychological state. Phrases such as 'having breathing space', 'waiting with baited breath' and 'it took my breath away' demonstrate the relationship between how a person *feels* and how their breath responds. Research tells us that airway and breathing patterns are affected by emotions. Patients with asthma are at least 50 per cent more likely than non-asthmatics to report anxiety, depression or alcohol dependence (Van Lieshout *et al.*, 2009). If birth is portrayed in movies or on TV, there is usually a supporter encouraging the labouring woman 'to breathe'. It is of benefit to know and share the evidence surrounding slow breathing with pregnant women and their partners. The emotional, psychological and physiological benefits are overwhelming.

A Swedish study in 2010 concluded that birth preparation with prophylaxis (relaxation techniques) showed no more beneficial effects on labour outcomes than standard education without prophylaxis. It was, however, associated with lower risk of emergency caesarean section, and more women were satisfied with the antenatal preparation than those with the standard care (Bergstrom, 2010). Another Swedish study (Waldenstrom and Irestedt, 2006) found that 92 per cent of women found psychoprophylaxis very effective and rated it as the most effective form of non-pharmacological pain relief. When assessing the effect of relaxation techniques taught in classes, the difficulty will always be data collection. Little evidence exists of the format of education for parents. There are midwives who will not be confident in leading a class through breathing techniques. If the facilitator has witnessed the benefits, and is confident in demonstration, the class will be receptive and more likely to use it. A conversation on breathing techniques is not enough to initiate practice, and use, in the parents.

Optimal breathing in a resting state mainly uses the diaphragm. Stress increases the breathing pattern and allows the ribcage to contribute to inspiration volume, resulting in thoracic breathing. Thoracic breathing is associated with increased dyspnoea (Courtney *et al.*, 2011). Rapid breathing is controlled by the sympathetic nervous system and is activated by stress. This type of breathing increases cortisol production and initiates the 'fight-or-flight' response. In contrast, slow breathing is a product of the parasympathetic nervous system.

Pranayama breathing is the practice of voluntary slow, deep breathing, consisting of a conscious inhalation, retention and exhalation. This breath work has been used for thousands of years in India. The East has long since recognised the importance of working with the breath. Martial arts, karate, Tai Chi and Chi Kung all have their foundation in breathing. There is recognition that the body is stronger with the breath. Any athlete will tell you that breath control is crucial. From tennis players and weight lifters to runners, they all use the breath to maximise their physical potential and strength.

A 2006 study revealed pranayama breathing to initiate the synchronisation of neural elements in the central nervous system, peripheral nervous system and surrounding tissues. It generates inhibitory signals by mechanically stretching tissues during breath inhalation and retention. This causes shifts in the autonomic balance towards parasympathetic dominance and results in a slowing of the heart rate and a relaxation of the sphincter muscles, including the cervix (Ravinder Jerath *et al.*, 2006). In another study looking at slow breathing over a period of 3 months, it was shown to improve autonomic function, while fast breathing had no effect on the autonomic nervous system (Pal *et al.*, 2004).

When examining the effects of slow breathing, and mental relaxation, on essential hypertension, a 2006 study yielded impressive results. It showed that even a single session of slow breathing, and mental relaxation, results in a temporary fall in blood pressure. With repetition, slow breathing was shown to produce a sustained reduction in blood pressure, heart rate and respiratory rate, while mental relaxation is more effective in reducing electromyographic activity and increasing peripheral skin temperature. The study recommended 10 minutes a day of slow breathing for long-term hypertension, to lower the complication rate and bring down the number and/or dosage of antihypertensive drugs (Kaushik *et al.*, 2006).

A 2003 study into the use of breathing techniques in asthma sufferers concluded that it can improve symptoms and reduce bronchodilator use (Cooper *et al.*, 2003). Further research conducted in 2008 has looked at the impact of initiating the relaxation response on gene expression. It revealed significant alterations in cellular metabolism that may counteract cellular damage related to chronic psychological stress (Dusek *et al.*, 2008).

In recent years the popularity of mindfulness has grown. This is a tool for recognising the mind–body continuum, reducing stress and increasing 'psychological flexibility' (Dunn *et al.*, 2012). The Oxford University NHS Trust, in collaboration with the University of Oxford Mindfulness Centre, introduced, in 2012, Mindfulness Based Childbirth and Parenting (MBCP). Preliminary results from the 9-week antenatal class have shown decreases in self-reported depression, perceived stress and anxiety, as well as significant personal benefits from undertaking the course. It is fast becoming acknowledged that mindfulness can have a profound impact on emotional, physical and psychological health. The Mindfulness in Schools Project (Kuyken *et al.*, 2012) executive summary states, 'there is good evidence from neuroscience and brain imaging that mindfulness meditation reliably and profoundly alters the structure and function of the brain to improve the quality of both thought and feeling'.

Mindfulness produces increased blood flow in the brain and a thickening of the cerebral cortex in areas associated with attention and emotional integration (Davidson, 2008). When the medical profession has been so long focused on Cartesianism, the ideology that the mind cannot improve the health of the body, a move towards Eastern philosophy, and the recognition of the mind–body connection, has forced a rethink towards health. These skills come under different headings: meditation, relaxation, mindfulness and yoga breathing, but all are proving to be more beneficial than we could have imagined, with far-reaching effects.

Breathing techniques can:

- reduce the stress response
- reduce blood pressure
- relax the sphincter muscles
- reduce oxygen consumption
- improve mental health
- reduce depression, and anxiety
- reduce physical pain
- alter brain structures
- increase physical energy.

Breathing for birth

Notice how small children breathe. Watch as their stomach moves with the breath. This is called diaphragmatic breathing.

On the inhalation breath, the stomach should rise slightly as the dome of the diaphragm contracts and compresses the abdominal space. On the exhalation, both the chest and the stomach fall. If you look at young children, this is what you usually see. In fact all mammals breathe diaphragmatically.

Now check your breathing. As adults we often breathe in and the chest rises as the intercostal muscles contract. When this happens, the stomach is drawn in. For women especially, we are very used to holding onto our abdominal muscles. Body image may impact on our ability to deep breathe. A flat stomach is seen as desirable, and therefore the breath has moved into shallow chest breathing. This is commonplace for many people. This type of breathing reduces the volume of oxygen available as it only partly expands the lungs. A normal thoracic breath draws only 500cc to 700cc of air in the average adult. This results in less efficient oxygen delivery to the circulatory system and subsequently less potential for physical action. A deep, abdominal breath typically draws 2,500cc to 3,000cc of air, expanding the entire lungs for optimal oxygen delivery (Jordan, 2014).

The hypnobirth breath can be called many things. The various 'brands' of hypnobirth will describe it as *surge breathing*, *birth breathing* or *up breathing*. These are all one and the same and are essentially diaphragmatic breathing. This is the breathing that the hypnobirthing woman will use throughout the first stage of labour.

The exercise below is used in a class to introduce breathing. It helps to engage the diaphragm and focus on the breathing, and allows the woman to become familiar with essential breathing for birth. You may want to try it for yourself:

- Lie on the floor face up with knees slightly bent. Place a small pillow under the head if that is more comfortable for you.
- Place your hands lightly on your stomach, your fingertips just touching.
- Concentrate on breathing using the diaphragm, not using the chest, and feel the stomach rise as the lungs fill from the bottom.

- As you breathe in, your fingertips should no longer touch.
- Let the stomach fall naturally when breathing out by relaxing the diaphragm.

The uterus in pregnancy is a large muscle. When a woman experiences a surge, the uterus becomes tight. If this tightness – the contracting – feels painful, the woman tenses. She may hold her breath. By doing so she is also tensing the abdominal wall which is covering the uterus. We now have two tight, tense, muscle layers, and muscle competition. Does it increase any pain? Yes. Surge breathing delivers extra oxygen to the uterus and the baby, relaxes the abdominal wall and releases tension. The surge becomes manageable.

Surge breathing practice

- Find somewhere comfortable and quiet to sit.
- Close your eyes and be mindful of your breath. Begin inhaling through the nose and, as you do, mentally, slowly, count to 3.
- As you exhale through the mouth, count to 6.
- Continue to breathe in, inflating the abdomen to a slow count of 3.
- Continue to breathe out, deflating the abdomen to a count of 6.
- You may notice a natural pause at the end of the out breath.
- Just rest in the space and wait for the in breath to come of its own accord.
- Inhale – 3.
- Exhale – 6.
- As you train your body to slow breathe, you may find your count changes. It may lengthen to 4 and 8, or even 5 and 10.
- Practice is the key!

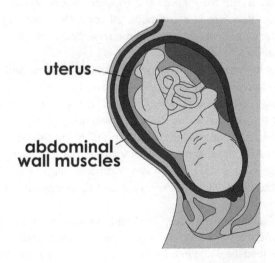

FIGURE 8.1 The uterus
Source: Lucy Martin

BOX 8.1 GRAHAM'S STORY

Where do we begin with the thank you?

We strongly believe that our experience would not have been possible had it not been for the support and guidance offered by you. The Hypnobirthing classes helped us both to understand the science behind the reality.

Our experience started on Friday afternoon. Kelly was booked in for her fourth and final sweep, prior to being induced. We desperately wanted to have a natural birth and the final sweep was our last chance. The thought of the induction did not scare us but we both felt that this would have robbed us of our experience. So the midwife came around 1.15pm; her words to Kelly were, 'let's get this baby out', certainly words that Kelly wanted to hear.

The midwife hadn't even got off our drive when Kelly started to experience surges, then putting into action all that we had been taught. I was advised to return home from work around 2.30pm. By the time I arrived home, Kelly was walking around the house breathing through the surges. I asked if she wanted to make her way to hospital but this was declined. The surges continued and so did Kelly's breathing, all throughout she had total control of the experience.

After speaking with the hospital at around 3.30 we decided that we should make our way to the hospital, as the surges were grouping nicely. The journey to the hospital was relaxed and calm; I won't lie, this was a surprise to me. Upon arrival at the MLU we were invited to our room, we made ourselves comfortable as the midwife chatted with Kelly regarding our surges. Upon examination we were 5cm, Kelly still breathing through the surges, totally in control, using minimal gas and air.

The surges started to become continuous, one after the other, after the other. We chatted with the midwife and thought that now may be the time to enter the pool. Kelly got into the pool, all the time breathing through the surges, with the occasional pep talk from me regarding controlling the breathing and occasional use of the gas and air.

For 4 hours Kelly experienced surges, breathing, moving and working with the surges. At approximately 8pm Kelly was asked if she wanted a final examination; this was agreed and Kelly was advised that she had escalated to 10cm. Bang on, just through controlling the breathing and shaking the apples in the pool. Kelly advised the midwife of our birthing plan and this was duly accepted. At approximately 8.30pm Kelly got back into the pool, the surges continuing, the midwife keeping a close eye on developments, all the while encouraging Kelly to breathe, along with me offering support to take control of the breathing and own it.

At around 9pm Kelly had birthed the head; we were invited to view. What an amazing experience: the mother-in-law saw baby looking around and wriggling, Kelly too confirmed the wriggling. The moment that we had both been so excited about was about to become a reality, we were going to have a baby.

The midwife asked me if I was ready to receive the baby. I was, nothing could have stopped me from receiving our baby and handing it to Kelly. I was a little nervous, but after looking into Kelly's eyes I knew everything was going to be ok. Kelly moved and I took the baby from her and, slowly, lifted it from the water to find out we had a baby girl. I handed her to Kelly, who, after all of her comments during the classes regarding the cleaning of the baby after birth, immediately kissed her. We were and are the proud parents of a healthy baby girl, Isla-Mai, and I couldn't be more proud of my wife, to show the strength and control through the birth, and I strongly believe that had we not done the hypnobirth classes this would have been a different story.

The whole experience was as rewarding as we wanted it to be and I would like to thank you from the bottom of my heart for assisting us throughout our pregnancy.

The myth of the push

Much has been debated around the subject of pushing. NICE recommend that women should be guided by their own instinctive urges during second stage. However, it has long been a cultural norm for the midwife to direct the woman to 'push'. This has often been accompanied by breath holding and 'pushing into your bottom'. This kind of directed pushing is called the valsalva manoeuvre. Holding the breath at this stage closes the glottis and has many disadvantages. Valsalva pushing reduces oxygen to the woman and the baby. It has been linked with increased perineal trauma and long-term effects on bladder and pelvic floor function.

From the many hundreds of women surveyed in antenatal classes, when women discuss second stage, there are common themes:

- How will I know when to push?
- Will the midwife tell me how to push?
- Will I poo?
- Will I tear?

The word 'push' encourages women to believe that at this stage they will actively move their baby some distance. There is a firm belief antenatally that a few 'pushes' will do it. As birth professionals, we know that second stage for many first-time women can take some hours. The myth of the push is misleading and deceptive. I like to describe second stage as 'nudging' the baby down. This may prepare the woman more accurately for the work involved and the time required. It is also worth discussing nudging with the breath. 'Pushing' has much historical context, and it seems impossible to view it in movies, and on TV, without the woman being told to hold her breath. It is often accompanied by instruction from the midwife, maybe with the partner joining in, often loudly. This consolidates the notion that women will need to be told when to push and undoubtedly will need instruction. By portraying birth in this way for so many years we have removed the woman from feeling that she is in any way the expert. Hypnobirth encourages women to work with the breath, and her body, for second stage. What we know is that a woman who is breathing her baby down, will instinctively nudge at the end of the breath. This is as it should be. Each woman is unique, and we cannot dictate how she will experience the surge, or what she should do with it.

There are various descriptions of second-stage breathing by the varying 'brands' of hypnobirth. You may hear it called *birth breathing*, *down breathing* or *J breathing*. These are all one and the same. J breathing makes sense as it describes visually the journey of the breath. It is describing the curve of the sacrum in the pelvis. Women have been used to diaphragmatic breathing in first stage. We now want them to send the breath lower, down into the pelvis, the pelvic floor and the vagina. You can try J breathing for yourself.

J breathing

This breathing is ALL through the nose:

- Take a breath in through your nose.
- Keeping your mouth gently closed, breath quickly down and visualise the 'J' shape of the pelvis.
- Send the breath down through your body and into the pelvic area.
- You should be able to feel a 'bulging' of the pelvic floor muscles.
- Repeat 3 times.

This type of breathing is not routinely practised in hypnobirth, but is encouraged for use on the toilet. When a bowel movement is required, J-breathing can assist by relaxing all the sphincter muscles. Katherine Graves describes this as taking a 'hypnopoo' and is definitely a term that parents relate to. Hypnopoos work well for everyone. You may want to try it!

Hypnobirth has an association with calm, peaceful birth. This can sometimes translate as silent. Of course we encourage a quiet birth environment, but the birthing woman is free to make noise, should she wish. Many of the hypnobirth DVDs shown in class portray women being very calm and quiet. This is in contrast to the screaming TV version of birth, but we have to be careful not to reinforce expectation of quiet birth. All women are different, and vocalisation in labour might be just what she needs. We practise using noise, with the breath, in class to allow women to see how it feels and sounds. Many physically challenging activities result in vocalisation. When practising martial arts, the karate noise is known as a kiai. Many Eastern philosophies believe that there is a force running through everything. This force is known as Ki in Japan or qi in China. Ki means energy, and ai means matching or uniting. Therefore kiai means working with the energy, something a labouring woman does beautifully. E. J. Harrison (1982), in his book *The Fighting Spirit of Japan*, describes it as the 'art of perfectly concentrating all one's energy, physical, and mental, upon a given object with unremitting determination so that one achieves one's goal'. This sentence can easily be applied to birth.

The kiai is used to ensure no breath holding; it focuses the mind and releases maximum energy. Many sportsmen, and women, use noise with the exhalation. Think of tennis players and weightlifters. Noise can be a powerful tool, and we do not want women to have a sense of failure if they use it. Hypnobirth is not silent. It is not Scientology. A calm birth does not always equate to a silent birth. If a woman grunts, sways, sweats and moans, she is still hypnobirthing!

References

Benson, H. (1975). The relaxation response. New York: Harper Collins.

Bergstrom, M. (2010). *Psychoprophylaxis – Antenatal preparation and actual use during labour.* Stockholm: Karolinska Institutet.

Cooper, S., Oborne, J., Newton, S., Harrison, V., Thompson Coon, J., Lewis, S. and Tattersfield, A. (2003). Effect of two breathing exercises (Buteyko and pranayama) in asthma: A randomised controlled trial. *Thorax*, 674–679.

Courtney, R., van Dixhoorn, J., Greenwood, K. M. and Anthonissen, E. L. M. (2011). Medically unexplained dyspnea: Partly moderated by dysfunctional (thoracic dominant) breathing pattern. *Journal of Asthma*, 259–265.

Davidson, R. L. A. (2008). Buddha's brain: Neuroplasticity and meditation. *IEEE Signal Processing Magazine*, 171–174.

Dunn, C., Haneih, E., Roberts, R. and Powrie, R. (2012). Mindful pregnancy and childbirth; Effects of a mindfulness based intervention on women's psychological distress and well being in the perinatal period. *Archives of Women's Mental Health*, 139–143.

Dusek, J.A., Out, H. H., Wohlhueter, A. L., Bhasin, M., Zerbini, L. F. and Joseph, M. G. (2008). Genomic counter-stress changes induced by the relaxation response. PLoS ONE.

Harrison, E. J. (1982). *The fighting spirit of Japan*. New York: Overlook Books.

Jordan, J. (2014, July 1st). Optimal method of breathing for martial arts training. Turtle Press: www.turtlepress.com/training/optimal-method-of-breathing-for-martial-arts-training. Retrieved September 25th 2015.

Kaushik, R. M., Kaushik, Reshma, Mahajan, Sukhdev Krishan and Rajesh, Vemreddi (2006). Effects of mental relaxation and slow breathing in essential hypertension. *Complementary Therapies in Medicine*, 120–126.

Kuyken, W., Weare, Katherine, Ukoumunne, Obioha C., Vicary, Rachael, Motton, Nicola, Burnett, Richard, Cullen, Chris, Hennelly, Sarah and Huppert, Felicia (2012). Effectiveness of the mindfullness in schools programme: non randomised controlled feasibility study. *The Br J Psychiatry*, 1–6.

Pal, G., Velkumary, S. and Madanmohan (2004). Effect of short-term practice of breathing exercises on autonomic functions in normal human volunteers. *Indian Journal of Medical Research*, 115–121.

Ravinder Jerath, J. W., Edry, Vernon A. and Barnes, Vandna Jerath (2006). Physiology of long pranayamic breathing: Neural respiratory elements may provide a mechanism that explains how slow deep breathing shifts the autonomic nervous system. *Med Hypotheses*, 566–571.

Van Lieshout, R. J., Bienenstock, J. and MacQueen, G. M. (2009). A review of candidate pathways underlying the association between asthma and major depressive disorder. *Psychosom Med*, 187–195.

Waldenstrom, U. and Irestedt, L. (2006). Obstetric pain relief and its association with remembrance of labor pain at two months and one year after birth. *Journal of Psychosomatic Obstet Gynecol*, 147–156.

9

HYPNOSIS FOR HYPNOBIRTH

All the hypnosis in hypnobirth is based on tried and tested techniques used by hypnotherapists. Hypnobirth in the NHS is taught by midwives who combine these techniques with the best antenatal education available. Once the hypnosis techniques have been learned, hypnobirth midwives are ideally skilled to teach the classes and to answer any medical questions that the couples may have.

Very few midwives, however, have experience in hypnotherapy, so the hypnosis techniques are specifically designed so that midwives can teach couples to become their own experts.

What is the difference between hypnosis and hypnotherapy?

The difference between hypnosis and hypnotherapy is that hypnotherapy includes therapeutic techniques as used by counsellors, psychotherapists or psychologists.

Although hypnobirth does not purport to be hypnotherapy, there is a simple, yet powerful, therapeutic technique that is used when doing the anxiety release exercise. It is a straightforward script that works well in a group setting. However, if any hypnobirth clients have mental health issues, and are undergoing medical treatment, they should consult their healthcare practitioner before doing this exercise in class. It may be appropriate to devise an individual care plan for them.

Of course, hypnobirth is designed to promote relaxation and calm, so it is an excellent programme to relieve stress and anxiety, for both mothers and their birthing partners.

Scripts

The purpose of hypnobirth scripts is to teach the mother the art of relaxation, which will then allow her to focus on her birth. Scripts can be broken down into their component parts and like all good stories they have a beginning, a middle and an end:

- induction
- deepeners
- guided visualisation
- emerge from hypnosis.

Induction of hypnosis

In hypnobirth, most scripts begin with an induction element. The first hypnobirth script that couples use is a progressive relaxation. This is the type of script that is often used at the end of a yoga session or an exercise class. The client will make herself comfortable and begin to relax her body, one bit at a time. This is a very gentle way to become relaxed and is easy for a woman, and her birthing partner, to use, as they begin to get into the habit of relaxing.

When someone begins to use hypnosis, they will often have thoughts like, 'I wonder if I'm hypnotised', 'I must get bread on my way home' or 'I forgot to phone so-and-so'. This is quite normal, so there is usually a sentence or two which mentions the thoughts that can drift in and out of the mind. The script explains that this is normal and offers a method of dealing with these occasional thoughts.

There is also a suggestion that any unexpected sounds will help the person to become more and more relaxed. Maternity units are not silent places, so it is important for women to be able to relax even when they can hear noises from other rooms, or people passing by. When working with a class it is useful to weave the sounds into the relaxation, for example if a you hear a nearby door bang, you might say: '... and every time you hear a door bang, you can allow yourself to become more and more relaxed ...'.

Sometimes when working with a group, in the middle of a relaxation, someone will come into the room unexpectedly. If this happens, we smile at them and make a 'shush-ing' gesture, and they will usually make an apologetic face and leave quietly. After the exercise has been completed, when asking the group if they noticed the interruption, most will say that they did not, and those that did will not have minded. This reinforces the message that, even birthing in a busy maternity unit, women can still achieve relaxation. Noises outside, midwives and students coming and going in the room, will not be disruptive. Both women and their partners can experience for themselves how hypnobirth takes them into 'the zone'.

With practice the mother will become more and more adept at relaxation, and when this happens there are shorter scripts where the induction is a simple instruction to relax. If the mother requires more practice, a short progressive relaxation can be added. It is essential to encourage couples to explore using the scripts, to make them their own. This means that they will be able to adapt to any circumstance that may arise; they will become their own hypnobirthing expert. Be mindful if you are caring for a hypnobirth couple that the birth partner will know what her triggers are for relaxation. They will have practised anchoring techniques, and he/she will be very aware of how to quickly relax the woman. Do ask for the partner's advice as you may be able to utilise these techniques too.

Breathing slowly is an important part of relaxation and, as the woman practises relaxation, and it becomes a habit, she can focus more and more on her breathing. These two activities combine to be the primary hypnobirthing tool that is used during surges. Hypnobirth midwives report that it can be difficult to tell when a hypnobirthing mother is experiencing a surge, because both her mind and body appear so relaxed.

BOX 9.1 PROGRESSIVE RELAXATION

[You may want to read the rest of this chapter, especially the section, 'Reading a script', before you start to read the script.]

Make yourself comfortable. Take a couple of nice deep breaths and, when you're ready, you can allow your eyes to gently close.

As you breathe in deeply and exhale slowly, you can allow yourself to relax ... breathing in deeply, exhaling slowly and, as you breathe out, you can allow your body to release ... relax ... just let go.

And as you begin to relax, you may become more aware of things around you ... the sounds in the room ... the sounds outside the room ... just allow all of these sounds to take you further and further into relaxation.

You may also become more aware of your thoughts ... things that you need to do ... but just take these few minutes for yourself now and allow your thoughts to drift in ... and out of your mind easily. And if any thoughts keep coming back into your mind, put them in a bubble and allow them to float away, just for now. As you listen to the sound of my voice and allow yourself to drift further and further into relaxation ... you can allow yourself to focus on what's important ... peace ... calm ... and relaxation.

Turning your attention to your head for a moment, allow a feeling of relaxation to develop in your head and face. Imagine the muscles of your scalp relaxing ... just by wanting it to happen it can happen.

Allow that feeling of relaxation to flow into your facial muscles now ... relaxing your forehead ... your eyebrows ... the tiny muscles around your eyes. Relaxing your cheeks. Relaxing your ears. Relaxing your mouth ... and your jaw ... relaxing your tongue.

You can allow this feeling of relaxation to flow down your neck ... relaxing your neck and throat ... flowing into your shoulders now ... releasing ... relaxing ... just let go. You can allow a lovely, warm feeling to flow with this feeling of relaxation ... softening and relaxing all of your muscles.

You can be interested to know whether this feeling of relaxation will move quickly or ... s-l-o-w-l-y down the arms now ... all the way down now ... all the way down, right the way down to very tips of your fingers. Soft, warm, gentle relaxation ... release ... relax ... just let go.

Allow that feeling to flow down your back, releasing ... relaxing the muscles on either side of your spine. Relaxing your chest, and allowing that feeling to flow down your body. Release ... relax ... just let go.

Now, allowing that feeling to flow through your hips into your legs. Relaxing your legs ... your thighs ... your shins and your calves. You can allow a feeling of heaviness to develop in your legs and the heavier they become, the more relaxed you can feel. The more relaxed you feel, the heavier they can become, allowing you to sink further and further into relaxation.

Now you can stay in this feeling of relaxation as long as you want. Resting in this space where time means nothing – an hour seems like a minute. A minute is just a blink. Rest in this space, relax ... relax ... relax.

[You can either move to the next part of the script, the deepener, or choose an emerge, to bring your subject out of hypnosis.]

Deepeners

Once the woman has begun to relax, the next step is to help her to go deeper and deeper. Deepeners are easy to follow, and usually have an element of predictability, which the client will find reassuring. Hypnobirth scripts often include counting backwards as a deepener, with the suggestion that, with every number, the subject will go deeper and deeper into relaxation; they will become more, and more, relaxed. Box 9.2 provides an example of a simple staircase deepener.

BOX 9.2 STAIRCASE DEEPENER

With your eyes closed, feeling comfortable ... in a moment you can begin to relax even further ... in a moment I'm going to begin counting backwards from 10 to 1.

When I say the number 10, you can imagine in your mind's eye that you are standing at the top of a flight of 10 stairs. Make your stairs safe and comfortable to walk down, perhaps there is a handrail.

As I say each number you will simply move down those stairs, relaxing more and more completely. At the bottom of the stairs is a path which you can walk along easily, calmly and comfortably. Even though you can't see exactly what's ahead of you along the path or around the corner you can be confident in your own ability and stay relaxed ... calm ... and comfortable.

When I say the number 1 you will step onto the path and take the first step of your journey.

So, breathe in deeply, and we can begin:

10 ... at the top of the stairs, you're relaxing and letting go;

9 ... becoming more relaxed, release ... relax ... just let go;

8 ... sinking into a more comfortable, peaceful and relaxed position;

7 You may notice sounds around you, simply allow these sounds to take you further and further into relaxation. Deeper and deeper, more and more relaxed;

6 ... way down now;

5 ... even further down;

4 ... you're doing perfectly ... deeper ... and deeper;

3 ... deeper ... and deeper;

2 ... more ... and more relaxed;

and 1 ... deeper ... and deeper ... more ... and more relaxed ... way down now.

That's fine, you're doing perfectly. Now walk along the path and take yourself to a beautiful place in nature and relax.

If you notice any sounds around you, this will allow you to relax even more. Deeper ... and deeper ... more ... and more relaxed.

[You can either move to the next part of the script, the guided visualisation, or pause for a few moments before you choose an emerge, to bring your subject out of hypnosis.]

Guided visualisation

The guided visualisation is simply the story that is told to encourage whatever resources are required. These may include: relaxation, confidence, peace, calm, tranquillity and anything else the mother may need. It usually involves asking the client to imagine a pleasant situation – e.g. walking along a path with beautiful flowers, or relaxing on a beach – and as she does, she is relaxing more and more. It may, of course, describe a scenario that the mother would like to rehearse.

It is important to make sure that your client is comfortable with the ideas that are about to be suggested. For example, if the visualisation includes a walk in a garden, it makes sense to ensure that no one in the group is frightened of or allergic to bees and other flying insects. Alternatively, simply make the suggestion that this garden is completely free of anything that may cause anxiety. It is also useful to include the suggestion that, wherever she is, it is perfect for her, and all she has to do is change anything that she does not like, to something that she does like.

Visualisation and imagery are an integral part of hypnobirth. The breathing techniques are linked to specific images that help mothers to stay focused and relaxed.

When couples become confident, they might adapt this portion of the script to include any resource that the mother might need and that has not already been included. Box 9.3 gives an example of a guided visualisation that anyone might find useful before embarking on a new challenge.

BOX 9.3 GUIDED VISUALISATION

Now, imagine yourself in this beautiful place, this beautiful place in nature ... perhaps it's warm ... make it the right temperature for you. Maybe you're beside some water ... a beautiful healing pool, with a waterfall. Make this place just right for you ... a place to rest, a place of healing, somewhere that feeds your soul, that makes your heart sing.

Provide yourself with everything you need to relax ... relax in this place and know that every time you come back here you can relax more deeply and more easily than before. Just by focusing on this place and taking a couple of deep breaths you can be transported into this feeling of relaxation.

And as you relax in this place, I'd like a part of you to come with me now. We're going to go on a journey. Follow the path once more and with every step you take you can become more and more relaxed ... with every step you take you can notice that you begin to enjoy this journey more ... and more. With every step you can feel more and more relaxed, as it becomes easier ... and easier.

And every time you take a step you can notice that your body feels lighter and lighter, almost as if you're floating. Your steps become lighter ... and lighter. And as you walk along you notice that you are coming to the edge of a tall cliff ... it's so tall it could even be the top of high mountain. And in a moment we're going to step off the mountain together, and fall down into the sky ... and allow ourselves to drift down ... and down ... ... and down. Remembering that you are in control and completely safe.

So take a deep breath and, as you take that step, you can allow yourself to drift down ... and down, floating now. Everything is calm and still ... everything is easy now. And there comes a moment that you realise you are no longer drifting, but that you are flying. You can allow the air currents, the wind, to support you effortlessly and weightlessly. As you feel all your cares and concerns flowing away ... resting in that space. Nothing else exists, just peace ... and calm ... and relaxation.

And as you rest in this feeling, I'd like a part of you to come with me now into the future and to see yourself a week from now. See yourself in a particular situation, it might be at work, or at home, but see yourself being more confident, more comfortable, happier. The changes may be small, just a week from now ... so go further into the future, a month from now. What can you see, in your mind's eye? Allow this to be the best possible future, allow yourself to imagine your innermost dreams and desires. See yourself acting 'as if'... whether that's at home or at work, notice the changes in your language, talking to your family, your friends and your colleagues.

Go further into the future now, a whole year from now and notice the changes ... the changes in you, and in the people around you, as you continue to make the changes that you want to make in your life. Make these changes the very best they can be. You can notice, perhaps, that you no longer have to act 'as if'; some of those changes are now the real you.

Now take a moment for the 'you in the future', to give the 'you of today' some good, useful advice, some practical hints and tips to help you to achieve all your hopes and dreams.

[Pause for a minute or so.]

In a moment it will be time to return to that beautiful place in nature, but before you do, say goodbye to the 'you of the future', just for now, give her (or him) a hug and thank her for her wisdom and advice.

Now find yourself back in that beautiful place, absorbing all those feelings of relaxation, feeling wonderful. And remember that, just by focusing on this place and taking a couple of deep breaths, you can be transported into this feeling of relaxation.

Now you can stay in this feeling of relaxation as long as you want. Resting in this space where time means nothing – an hour seems like a minute. A minute is just a blink. Rest in this space, relax … relax … relax ….

[Now choose an emerge and bring your subject out of hypnosis.]

Emerge from hypnosis

In hypnobirth scripts, the client will usually emerge from hypnosis slowly. The suggestion is often made that they bring their attention back into the room at their own pace. The longer it takes, the more relaxed they know they have been. This helps clients to trust in themselves, and in the techniques.

The gradual emerge from hypnosis works perfectly in labour, where the mother is in control of her level of relaxation. A well prepared birthing partner will be attuned to her hypnobirth skills and will encourage her, and guide her when appropriate.

BOX 9.4 SLOW EMERGE FROM HYPNOSIS

In a moment it will be time to come back into the room, feeling confident and relaxed, knowing that each time you do this you will find it easier and easier to relax, and you will feel more and more confident. So you can begin by moving your fingers and toes, take a nice deep breath and, in your own time, you can gently open your eyes, feeling great.

[Then leave them to come to, in their own time.]

A quicker emerge is included in some scripts; these are more akin to the suggestions made in a clinical setting. If a woman should need to be brought out of hypnosis quickly, these can be used and she will be familiar with them. It can feel very disorientating to startle someone from a deeply relaxed state of hypnosis, and it should be avoided unless absolutely necessary.

BOX 9.5 QUICKER EMERGE FROM HYPNOSIS

[This is read a little more briskly in order to bring your subject out of hypnosis more quickly.]

In a moment I'm going to count from 1 up to 5 and, on the count of 5, you can open your eyes, feeling calm, confident and relaxed. Feeling really great, knowing that each time you do this you will find it easier and easier to relax, and you will feel more and more confident.

1. ... beginning to become aware of your surroundings ...
2. ... take a nice deep breath ...
3. ... your eyelids are feeling lighter ...
4. ... your hands are beginning to move ...
5. ... eyes open, return to the room feeling relaxed and confident, feeling great.

Reading a script

Now that you have all the elements for a script, you can try it for yourself. You may want to put on some relaxing music and read it to a friend or colleague, or get them to read it to you.

Sometimes hypnotherapists will use a rather sing-song voice, this may make you feel very self-conscious, which will come through to the person who is listening and will be unlikely to be relaxing. It is more likely that they will find it a bit weird! So keep your voice normal, just read very slowly and, as you relax, you can find your voice becoming softer and gentler.

The important thing to remember, when reading a script, is to read it very slowly. You will notice gaps in the text, and sometimes the grammar can seem a little different from normal speech, but just read it as it is written. If you make a mistake, just keep going. Even though you will think you are reading very slowly, you can read it much more slowly than that!

Post-hypnotic suggestions

Post-hypnotic suggestions are used to encourage hypnobirthing women to practise the techniques and to reinforce the skills that they will learn. For example:

'Allowing yourself to come back into the room, feeling confident and alert, knowing that every time you practise this you will find it easier and easier, and you'll be able to go deeper and deeper into relaxation ...' or,

'When you feel your partner's hand touch you, or you hear your partner's voice, you feel calm, and relaxed.'

It is good practice to keep the couples for at least 10 minutes after a script reading; they will still be very open to suggestion. It is important to keep talking in a positive way, which will reinforce the work that they have just been doing. It also prevents others from undoing that great work.

There are other techniques that are taught in hypnobirth that are included within the scripts. These are:

- reframing
- anchors and triggers
- matching and pacing.

Reframing

We have talked a lot about the effect of language. Reframing is a brilliant technique that supports the use of positive language, thoughts and statements. In its simplest form it is taking a 'glass-half-empty' thought and turning it into a 'glass-half-full' one. This is a Neuro Linguistic Programming (NLP) technique and is not hypnosis, but can be used under hypnosis to make a positive reframe. It is also a powerful way to train yourself, or another, to think positively. Birth partners are important reframers and will be able to assist the woman to change any negative thoughts around birth.

Exercise: When you are at work, notice the language that is used around you and think about the impact that it could have on a pregnant couple. Are you speaking to them in a medicalised way? Do they appear to be uneasy or confused? Think about how you can put them at ease with the words that you use. One of the most important uses of reframing is when you notice yourself using negative phrases, and thoughts, and you become adept at reframing them at the time. This will produce a positive result, not just for you but for the couples that you support.

The reframing techniques used in most hypnobirth methods are very similar. They are usually under the heading 'Fear Release' or 'Anxiety Release'. The first step is to ask the couples to think about all the things that they are worried about. This might be an event from the past, a previous birth experience, perhaps. It may be something in the future that is making them anxious. This exercise is not just for mothers, it is for anyone who will be attending the birth. Anxiety can be contagious; it is very difficult for a mother to relax, if the birthing partner is pacing up and down anxiously. If a woman catches a nervous look passed between two midwives, it can be enough to bring her out of her relaxed space and to halt her production of oxytocin.

Once the couple has made a list of their anxieties, they should sit down together and discuss them. It has often been the case that the mother is worried about very pragmatic issues. For example:

- getting to the hospital, especially in the winter months when the roads might be icy;
- finding a babysitter in the night for their young toddler.

Sometimes the response from the birth partner has been, 'I've thought about that, and this is what we'll do …'. Once they begin to discuss the list of anxieties, it becomes possible to find a solution and cross them off the list.

If the anxiety is about the birth, this may have been caused by external stories, things she has seen on TV, traumatic birth stories told by her friends or family, or she may feel out of control because this is a new experience. The technique used in class is to change this picture while in hypnosis; this helps to release the anxiety, or fear, and create a calm and empowering picture of the future.

The important thing to remember is that it is not an event that causes the problem, but how a person feels about it. Two people can have a similar experience but have very different feelings about it. Most negative feelings occur when the person feels powerless; the negative feelings come from the way that others behaved towards that person, and especially the language that they used.

If a mother has experienced a difficult birth, she may need to do this exercise more than once. She could do this at home with her birth partner, or she might prefer to find a therapist who can help her with trauma release. Her birth partner may also have some trauma that he or she needs to work on.

Triggers and anchors

Triggers are very powerful. When someone wants to change an unwanted behaviour, it is important to identify the actions that trigger this particular habit. For smokers, there are lots of common triggers, e.g. when the telephone rings; after a meal; or with a glass of wine. So, when breaking a habit such as smoking, identifying the triggers and changing them in even a small way can help the process. I overheard a conversation recently between a young woman who is in the process of becoming a non-smoker and a man who has been a non-smoker for several years now.

She said: 'I'm doing really well, except when I'm at work. If someone else goes outside for a cigarette, I really want to go with them. But I don't smoke at all when I'm at home – I don't even think about it.'

He responded: 'I really struggled when I used to go out to the pub for a drink. So I stopped going for a while until I had cracked it, and now I can have a beer without wanting a cigarette, it's great!'

We know that stress and anxiety are unwanted during labour because they can lead to the stress–tension–pain cycle. We also want to avoid stress and anxiety during pregnancy in order to create a calm environment for the baby to develop. This is why we ask couples to avoid listening to negative birth stories, whether that's from family and friends or television soaps, dramas or documentaries. It is also why it is important to practise their relaxation as much as possible to counteract the normal day-to-day stresses.

Exercise: Triggers can also be used in a positive way: to remind us to do a task. Perhaps you can think of a few triggers that you'd like to implement for yourself – you can write them here:

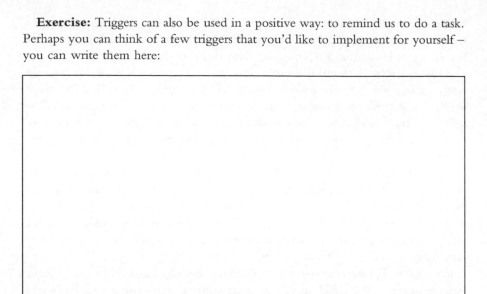

Anchors are physical cues to a feeling of relaxation or to strengthen a particular suggestion. They are simple and easy to use. Anchors can be used in all sorts of situations; every time a certain situation occurs, it will trigger a particular feeling or action. For example, when a client is in a state of deep relaxation, the suggestion can be made that, every time her partner touches her on the shoulder and applies a gentle downward pressure, she will become twice as relaxed. The anchor helps the client to remember the detail of the suggestion when she needs it the most. This is especially effective in childbirth.

Matching and pacing

Matching and pacing is a technique that can be used to take someone from one state into a different state. First you must match the state that they are in and then gradually move into the state that you would like them to be in. Here are some examples.

I was recently in a hotel reception where a customer was extremely unhappy with the service he had received. The receptionist said something that was clearly the final straw, and the man exploded into angry shouting, which ended with the manager being called. The customer continued to shout his displeasure, and at first the manager also spoke in quite a loud voice. Very quickly the manager slowed the pace of his speech and reduced the volume, and within a short space of time the angry customer began to calm down. He then apologised for his outburst and was willing to listen to the manager, who did his best to rectify the problem.

Another wonderful example of using matching and pacing to good effect was a story told to me by a midwife. She was caring for a woman whose labour was going quite slowly, and it was close to the time frame set by the hospital. A doctor came into the room demanding to know why this woman had not already been put on a drip. He was rather loud, and brusque, and was interrupting the calm relaxation in the room.

The midwife smiled at the doctor and then turned to the woman and began to talk to her in a calm voice, suggesting that she take some long slow breaths, that she notice herself become more and more calm. She continued in this way for several minutes during which time the doctor's hands had dropped to his sides, his breathing had slowed and his state of mind had changed. He then said that perhaps she could be left a little longer as all seemed to be well and he left the room. The woman went on to birth her baby naturally.

We can see from this that it is possible to influence others indirectly with calm breathing and gentle words.

On another occasion, a father reported to me that a doctor had come into their room with much the same attitude and, when asked if he had read their birth plan, the doctor answered that he had not. The father suggested that he go and read it, and come back again later. The doctor left the room and did not return. They went on to have a calm birth even though it was rather slow. This is a great example of a hypnobirth father who was confident, calm and empowered.

Self-hypnosis

An expression that is often used by hypnotherapists is that all hypnosis is self-hypnosis; this is undoubtedly true of hypnobirth. The couples learn the hypnosis techniques from their hypnobirth midwife and practise them until they become experts for themselves.

10

CAN YOU LOW RISK THE HIGH RISK?

As we have conceded that hypnobirth is growing in popularity, it would be wise to accept that many hypnobirth couples will not meet the low-risk criteria and will birth their babies in an obstetric unit. A hypnobirth can be achieved in all locations, but it can seem that the obstetric area represents some challenges for hypnobirthing couples. It could be argued that the woman experiencing intervention is the one who will benefit most from relaxation techniques. There sometimes feels like a gulf between obstetrics and midwifery, but the two can intertwine beautifully. *Obstetrix* was originally the Latin word for 'midwife'; it is thought to derive from *obstare* (to 'stand before'), because the attendant stood in front of the woman to receive the baby. Only in the twentieth century did the subject taught in medical schools change its name from 'midwifery' to 'obstetrics', perhaps because a Latin name seemed more academic than the Anglo-Saxon, derived from *mid*, 'with', and *wyf*, 'woman' (APA, 2015).

Risk

We have already discussed the importance and impact of language. However, early on in pregnancy we label the woman as high risk or low risk. We never talk about no risk. Risk assessment as a healthcare provider is a continuum – it is constantly being reassessed and updated. In her 2010 reflection on risk assessment, Sara Wickham raises the issue of gaining informed consent to formally risk assess the woman. She argues that the woman's risk status will affect the woman's choices and care, and therefore should be made with consent. She also talks about formal, and informal, risk assessment. Formally, we measure and record the level of risk. Informally, as healthcare providers, we make judgements. How often have you heard descriptions in the handover room that have nothing to do with the clinical picture?

When a risk assessment is performed, and the woman has been satisfactorily labelled, the information regarding the risk should be discussed. The word 'risk' is an emotive one. It is a word that many women do not wish to hear in association with their pregnancy and baby. Once it has been said, it will be difficult to relieve the anxiety it brings. What many women fail to understand, and to be told, is what the *actual* risk is. Sentences that are not acceptable, but often used, include:

- You are at greater risk of bleeding.
- You double your chances of having a still birth.
- There is a risk of your placenta failing.

If a risk is being described as doubling, the woman needs to know actual percentages. If the risk doubles from 0.0002 per cent to 0.0004 per cent, she might find that an acceptable risk. If it doubles from 25 per cent to 50 per cent, she may find that unacceptable. Unfortunately there is much fast and loose talk surrounding risk, with little solid evidence. If the risk has an impact on her birth choices, she should have all the information, including the risk of iatrogenesis, and not just the bit we choose to share. We often discuss informed consent within the medical profession, implying that, however much information is shared, the eventual outcome will be consent. Levy's (1999) research describes how the framing of information shapes choice profoundly. She uses the term, 'gently steering' to capture how the midwives and medics coax women to choices that they are comfortable with. Lothian (2008) argues that women's choices are limited by physicians and hospitals. She uses examples such as limiting the number of birth supporters, eating and drinking in labour, the availability of birth pools, birth balls and alternative equipment. She goes on to say, 'Choice is further limited by the withholding of information or providing information to women that is consistent with restrictive hospital rules and obstetricians' protocols rather than with evidence-based information.'

Normality

'We use the term normal birth to mean labour and birth without medical interventions. Other ways we might refer to this are natural birth, physiological birth or straightforward vaginal birth' (BirthchoiceUK, 2012).

Is it possible to reframe the impact that labels have on women's perception of their pregnancy? Once a pregnancy has been labelled high risk, it can be difficult for the woman (and some practitioners) to find the normality within the high risk.

When influential institutions such as The National Institute for Health and Care Excellence place childbirth under the heading of 'condition and disease', it would seem a lost cause. As midwives, we spend a lot of time reinforcing to women that pregnancy is not an illness and that birth is a normal life event and can happen at home. However, our literature and information does not support this. Medicalisation can be an interactive process, and Wertz and Wertz (1989) point out that pregnant women are actively involved in the medicalisation of their own pregnancy and birth. There will always be women who feel pregnancy to be an abnormal state. For some women, pregnancy worsens co-morbidities. However women feel, childbirth is under medical surveillance, and this has expanded over the decades to include the antenatal and postnatal periods and infertility. Davis-Floyd (1992) notes that the simple fact that a woman enters hospital to birth indicates that she holds categories in her mind that correspond to the technocratic model. At every antenatal appointment we discuss with the woman 'normality' and encourage normal birth. This normal birth discussion happens early on. Even whilst reassuring her that everything is 'normal', we are measuring her fundus, monitoring her blood pressure, dipping her urine, taking her blood and recording the findings using words she may not understand. We have reduced the woman to a set of numbers and assessed her ability to birth her baby long before the event. She then has 40 weeks to mull over her chances of success.

The implications of defining a pregnancy and birth as normal have massive ramifications, as the alternative to this is abnormal. Is normal low risk? Is high risk abnormal? The conflicting messages that women receive place doubt and fear in their minds. If she did not give birth 'normally' first time around, was it abnormally?

Research conducted by Green (1993) into birth expectation revealed that women tended to get what they expected in labour. If they expected pain, then this was realised in the birth room. Women who used breathing and relaxation techniques, and expected them to work, did so successfully. If a woman is labelled high risk from the outset, and the expectation is one of intervention, evidence tells us she will adjust her mindset to conform to this. She will no doubt oblige with the birth that the establishment has forecast for her.

Normal birth must be a belief system that is upheld by the care giver, the organisation, society, the woman and her supporting family for it to be made a reality. Although we pay lip service to the holy grail of normality, it can feel further and further away from the everyday reality of the labour ward. The medicalisation of childbirth has given rise to a 'natural birthing' movement: midwifery-led units, the National Childbirth Trust, doulas, the Active Birth movement, hypnobirth and freebirthing. However, it has not resulted in the demedicalisation of childbirth. It is still defined as a medical event. When so many women continue to opt for a hospital birth, the undercurrent in society suggests that birth is a medical event and best performed in the hospital.

Schmid (2011) suggests a move towards a health paradigm, where the focus switches from pathology to health, with the assumption of normality. Could the default location for birth be home, switching to a hospital birth when indicated in pregnancy?

Allowing the not allowed

What are our attitudes to women who will not allow the not allowed? When we meet the woman who has experienced three caesarean births and wants number four at home? The woman with twins, who wants a pool rather than an epidural? These are often women who have thought very carefully about their choices and outcomes. Rejecting the medical model can be a direct result of a previous experience, and the establishment has to accept that, for whatever reason, it made her feel this way. It often does not and labels her as difficult. When a woman takes responsibility for her care, it can shift the power. Within a patriarchal institution this can cause a well-known phenomenon – playing the dead baby card. Dagustun (2012) describes it as an 'acknowledged and accepted part of medical culture, used to gain control over childbirth decision-making'.

For some women a normal birth experience may just happen. For others it is fought for, a proactive journey with birth preparation, birth plans and an equal voice during labour. There are many factors that can influence a woman's birth outcome. The obvious influences – health and well-being in pregnancy, good support during labour, relaxation techniques, continuity of care and expectations around pain – all tend to be discussed. The covert influences are more difficult to address. The midwife's attitude towards pain, the labour ward culture, the politics and dynamics of the particular Trust, the variation in Trust guidelines and the professional's interpretation of the guideline. What is apparent is that the health professional in the birthing room can influence the labour and outcome dramatically.

Intervention – the hypnobirth perspective

VEs

Ways of assessing the progress in labour have been debated since Emanuel Friedman (1954) recorded cervical dilatation and produced the Friedman curve. Organisational factors in today's busy obstetric units result in birth being measured in terms of progress and not process. Later research (Albers, 1999) provided evidence that labours were longer than Friedman had concluded, sometimes twice the length. Walsh (2012) suggests that the increase in general health of women now, compared with 50 years ago, makes them more likely to cope with longer labours. Zhang et al. (2002) rationalise that a mean increase in maternal and fetal weight is probably contributing to slower labours. The study revealed the cervix dilated substantially more slowly in the active phase, taking approximately 5.5 hours from 4cm to 10cm, compared with 2.5 hours under the Friedman curve. On the basis of Zhang's work, Walsh (2012) suggests that active labour for some women, regardless of parity, starts between 5cm and 6cm dilatation. There is a shift in understanding that labour progress should not be determined by cervical dilatation alone. However, linear notions of labour progress are still prevalent. The weight of importance attached to the vaginal examination (VE) is reflected on the labour ward's white board. A missing VE will often result in an array of questions as to why it has not been performed. Vaginal examinations are invasive, and the procedure alone is enough for many women to produce catecholamines. This production of stress hormones will result in reduced blood flow to the uterus, reducing, and slowing, the efficiency of uterine contractions. Blood flow to the fetus is reduced, labour is then delayed. (Davies, 2011).

Midwifery skills for assessing the process of labour without performing a VE include recognition of the purple line. This line stretches from the anal margin and extends between the buttocks as labour progresses. Shepherd *et al.* (2010) found that an incidence of 76 per cent of women displayed the line. The sample was small, 144 women, but identified a positive correlation between the length of the line and cervical dilatation. Edmonds and Byrne (1990) reported that 89 per cent of women developed the line. Hobbs (1998) observes that the line does not seem to rise in strict proportion; there is a longer gap between 4cm and 7cm dilatation than there is both before and after. However, she does support the accuracy of the line.

Anne Frye (2004) suggests recognising temperature changes on the surface of the mother's leg between the ankle and the knee. Most, but not all, women experience a temperature change in their calf when they labour. When the woman is not yet dilated, the toes and feet may be cold, but the rest of the leg is warm. As labour progresses, the line of demarcation between the cold region and the warm region moves up the leg from the ankle towards the knee. When the entire calf is cold, but the knee is warm, full dilatation has been reached.

Other skills for assessing the process could include abdominal palpation, the frequency and pattern of uterine surges and anal dilatation. Downe *et al.* (2013) summarised a Cochrane review into vaginal examinations:

> It is surprising that there is such a widespread use of this intervention without good evidence of effectiveness, particularly considering the sensitivity of the procedure for the women receiving it, and the potential for adverse consequences in some settings. The effectiveness of the use and timing of routine vaginal examinations in labour, and other ways of assessing progress in labour, including maternal behavioural cues, should be the focus of new research as a matter of urgency. Women's views of ways of assessing labour progress should be given high priority in any future research in this area.

Top tips for VEs

- The National Institute for Health and Care Excellence (NICE, 2014) state that all women should be offered a VE every 4 hours.
- Be aware that some women will choose to decline the offer of a VE or postpone it to a time when they feel ready.
- NICE (2014) also says 'be sure that the examination is necessary and will add important information to the decision-making process'.
- The VE should be performed between surges if possible.
- Encourage the woman to use her hypnobirth breathing – the more relaxed she is, the easier and quicker it will be.
- Midwives can examine women whilst they are in the birth pool.

- Once the VE is complete, make sure the woman returns to an upright comfortable position.
- Consider other ways to assess dilatation.

Caesarean birth

The hypnobirth couple will have planned for a normal birth, but understand that intervention can be necessary. When birth moves to surgery it will be their relaxation skills that improve a difficult experience.

BOX 10.1 CAROLYN AND MICHAEL'S STORY

The hypnobirthing classes really helped us through the whole experience, which didn't quite go to plan.

On Tuesday I went into pre-labour at home, by the evening surges were 3 minutes apart. As I was comfortable at home using the breathing techniques, on contacting the birth unit they advised that I stayed at home at that time.

On Wednesday the surges had continued and remained 3 minutes apart but were longer in duration; that evening the birth unit asked me to go in. On examination, I was 5cm dilated and agreed to continue with my breathing next to the birthing pool. We created a lovely nest with a pre-made music playlist, candles, starlit ceiling, and we had lots of snacks and felt quite relaxed. After 8 hours I was 7cm and agreed to use the birthing pool with my green B&Q knee pads at the ready!

I had a further examination after 4 hours of being in the pool to find that I was 9cm, at this point only using gas and air. I re-entered the pool for a further 2 hours; however, I stayed at 9cm, so my waters were broken (now it's the 24th September).

This is when the situation got complicated as I had a significant amount of meconium in my waters. I was taken through to a delivery room where I spent a further 2 hours having surges, only to find I was still 9cm and the baby in a difficult position, not moving down.

As a result of being tired, I agreed to have an epidural and to be placed on a hormone drip to increase the surges. Unfortunately I had to wait for the epidural, which is when the breathing techniques were most helpful and allowed me to remain in some control. While having the epidural I was experiencing the most intense surges imaginable and needed to remain extremely still – this was only made possible by my learning from hypnobirthing.

After a further 2 hours of the hormone drip I achieved 10cm; however, the baby had not moved position and remained not moving down the birth canal. I tried pushing for another 1.5 hours with no success and was then told that the baby was in distress.

Forceps was discussed; however, on review a consultant decided an emergency C-section was needed to take place straight away. I was rushed through to theatre with me and Michael now both using the hypnobirthing breathing exercises. I was able to stay calm and breathe while having my anaesthetic in my back, despite being extremely distressed myself. The C-section was very traumatic, as Erin was born not breathing and needed to be resuscitated; after what seemed to be forever we heard her cry. She spent the night in the high-risk unit having one-to-one care; we got to meet her properly in the morning and she was allowed onto the ward with me the night of the 25th due to progress in her condition.

Hypnobirthing continued to be useful in the 9 days that followed, as we both were ill and not fit for discharge. Erin and I had an infection and I was diagnosed with maternal sepsis. To top it off I also was found to have heart problems. Erin had to have a number of tests including a lumbar puncture and blood tests; she had a cannula throughout our stay in hospital which was very stressful and resulted in the golden thread visualisation being visited almost daily! I have a phobia of wrists and needed to have a blood test from my arteries for oxygen levels and another cannula fitted – I think I used every single technique we learnt over this time!

I am happy to say we were discharged on the 2nd October, with Erin making a full recovery after two courses of antibiotics. The staff at the hospital were truly amazing: they were reassuring, calming and caring. We are incredibly grateful for their knowledge and skills. Without them we know things would be very different. It was not only them doing their job which touched us but that they were so caring also. For example: Michael left theatre to be with Erin; at this time the anaesthetist offered to hold my hand, another person was talking to me about cooking, who was very funny, discussing brownies. The consultant spoke to us throughout the whole C-section to keep us updated and, even when giving bad news, was reassuring. Michael was allowed to spend the night with me in the delivery room, being given a bed next to me and was allowed to shower the next morning before we were able to see Erin. Erin was brought to us that night from high risk for 5 mins for skin on skin before being taken back to the unit. The two midwives offered to take a number of family photos and photos of me with Erin, which was so special. We could say so much more about the personal and professional service that we received that cannot be faulted.

We feel that, without hypnobirthing, our ability to stay calm and cope would have been significantly impacted, which would have made the situation so much worse. Even through the worst time of our lives we stayed focused and determined to assist the process in whatever way we could.

Thank you for everything, your enthusiasm on the course allowed us to enjoy and retain our learning, which was of benefit to the birth of our beautiful daughter Erin Scarlett.

Hypnobirth couples may plan an elective caesarean birth, in which case we can implement some of the tips below:

- When discussing the woman's caesarean, substitute the word 'birth' for 'section'. It will make her feel better. She is giving birth after all.
- Before the birth there is often a wait. The surge breathing techniques can be used to keep her calm and relaxed.
- Birth partners can use three-step touch breathing during this time.
- Play the hypnobirth CD in the wait before birth. It could also be played in theatre.
- Use a tissue and place a drop of her favourite relaxing aromatherapy oil on it. (She may have used it to relax to at home, so it will be a trigger.) Give it to the birth partner to put into the pocket of their scrubs. This can be used during the birth – a quick sniff will be a trigger for relaxation.
- Offer for the drape to be lowered at the moment of birth.
- Anchors such as a shoulder anchor are popular with woman experiencing a caesarean birth.
- The birth partner may want to read a short script, or use a hypnosis induction technique.
- Ask if they know the sex of the baby and, if not, do they wish to discover it for themselves? The drape lowering moment may be ideal for this.
- Can you facilitate delayed cord clamping? Even 30 seconds longer is beneficial to the baby, and the parents will know this.
- Skin-to-skin contact should be initiated immediately after birth. If this is not possible for some reason, then skin to skin with the birth partner.
- Baby to be weighed only after prolonged skin to skin and with the mother in the room. Place the baby tummy down in the scales. This is an instinctive fetal position for baby and causes less distress.
- Suggest probiotics post-natally.

Emerging research shows that bacteria are absolutely vital for human health, and imbalances in the human microbiome significantly contribute to chronic non-transmissible diseases. The microbiome is gut bacteria that is cultured during the vaginal birth process. The baby is 'seeded' as it passes through the birth canal. Babies born by caesarean birth have a third less bacteria variety than babies born vaginally. This can affect their long-term health. The documentary, *Microbirth* (www.microbirth.com) explains how women experiencing a caesarean birth can reproduce the optimum gut flora, and this is growing in popularity with women and their partners. We will see more women asking for their baby to be 'seeded'.

At least an hour before birth, the mother inserts a sterile gauze that has been soaked in normal saline into the vaginal birth canal. The gauze needs to be folded like a concertina, with lots of surface area. This will culture the trillions of bacteria that are usually passed to the baby during birth. The sterile gauze is removed just before birth and kept in a sterile container. Once the baby is birthed, the gauze is used to wipe the baby's face, nose, mouth and rest of the body (the parents can do this, or the midwife). Although this practice may seem a little 'alternative', just as waterbirth and hypnobirth seemed alternative, it will gain credence and popularity. Women and their partners are knowledgeable and well educated on the benefits and risks of caesarean birth. If their pregnancy results in a necessary caesarean birth, there are some health elements they feel they can take back. Seeding the baby, delayed cord clamping and skin to skin are all involved in adding value to a birth that may have not been their first choice.

BOX 10.2 ARCHANA AND VINIT'S STORY

We started the programme planning a normal delivery but then mid-way we opted for an elective C-section and we were positively surprised by how useful the programme was even for C-sections. We must also note that the ability to quickly refocus the programme mid-way was remarkable.

What we found most useful was the really relaxed state we achieved thanks to hypnobirthing in all the three stages in the days before our operation date; on the day when we waited for the operation; and even during the surgery.

In the run up to the surgery, I noticed the biggest impact on my wife was her sleeping improved dramatically, as we were practising the relaxation techniques at bed time. This had a very calming effect on her as, prior to hypnobirthing, her sleep was quite disturbed.

On the day, we carried the music on my phone and listened to it as we waited for our turn. That reduced the stress significantly.

During surgery our level of relaxation was visible in our constantly updating our friends and family back home using social networking, clearly a visible measure of success of the programme.

Further, post-delivery, I even agreed to cut the cord, something I would never have thought I would get myself to do.

Our baby was born healthy, but with a cut behind his ear and, again, the relaxed state of mind achieved from hypnobirthing went a long way to help as the baby slowly healed.

I use these relaxation techniques even now, 1 month after delivery, and in fact have come to believe that these are of immense use even in our day-to-day lives.

Induction of labour

What a shame women are handed a piece of paper with an 'estimated delivery date' printed on it. Most women immediately knock off the word 'estimated' and, from that moment forward, the expectation has been set. If women themselves believe pregnancy to be 'overdue' at 41 weeks, then we can only blame ourselves for setting them up to fail. Induction of labour is increasing rapidly in the UK. Questions need to be asked about its use and effectiveness. If not questioned,

I believe we will see an induction rate in line with the caesarean birth rate before long. More frequently we are supporting women who are fit and well but at 42 weeks have yet to give birth. For those women with co-morbidities it is often wholly appropriate to induce labour. But here we are discussing the straightforward pregnancy.

The normal–abnormal continuum can be seen clearly with prolonged pregnancy. Between 37 and 42 weeks the woman fits the normal continuum. She experiences midwife-led care, the birth environment is seen as central and covert risk assessment is performed. She is regarded as an individual and within social context. This is normal for her. At 42 weeks plus a day the continuum shifts to abnormal. She now experiences obstetric-led care. The birth environment is peripheral, choice is limited. Risk assessment is overt and this is no longer normal for her, but normal for the establishment. Her individuality is limited by her gestation. Although for us, as healthcare professionals, this is a normal journey, for the woman, the switch is sudden and dramatic.

The World Health Organization states that induction of labour (IOL) should be performed only when there is a clear medical indication for it and the expected benefits outweigh its potential harms (WHO, 2011). Studies by Lewis *et al.* (1975) and Kitzinger (1978) reveal that women felt unprepared for IOL and lacked information. NICE guidance states that women should be given information on the induction process at 38 weeks of pregnancy. At 38 weeks of pregnancy many women are anticipating the birth they have planned. As we know the importance of the power of language and expectation, discussing intervention at this stage can cause anxiety and stress. An Australian study concluded that women booked for induction felt unprepared for their shift in birth expectations and lacked information (Gatward *et al.*, 2010).

Westfall and Benoit (2004) documented the feelings of isolation and the increased need for support in women who were approaching term pregnancy and wished to avoid induction.

Women booked for induction are associated with increased risk of anxiety or depression compared with women awaiting spontaneous labour (Cartwright, 1979). Many women at this stage experience dividing emotions. They feel committed to achieving the hypnobirth they had planned and have been using affirmations to believe their bodies are strong and competent. And yet by 41 weeks it is being suggested that their baby and body are not competent and that the medical profession knows best.

Studies by Uvnas-Moberg *et al.* (2005) demonstrate how a woman can respond to stimuli or situations where she feels threatened or anxious. Catecholamines, epinephrine and norepinephrine are released in preparation for the 'fight-or-flight' stress response. Studies into the effects of adrenalin on mammalian pregnancy reveal that stress can influence fetal growth, placental morphology, preterm labour or fetal death in some species (Naaktgeboren, 1979). High catecholamine levels in late pregnancy inhibit the production of oxytocin. This therefore inhibits the likelihood of labouring spontaneously.

There are many risks associated with IOL, many of which are not discussed with the woman. The woman can experience a shift in expectation, and therefore a loss of her birth plan. Many inductions take place on an antenatal ward and she will face the possibility of loss of support, if she is not labouring, and her partner is asked to go home. The medical environment produces a surplus of adrenalin, and she faces exogenic oxytocin production rather than endogenic. She may experience feelings of failure, her birth and her body having been medicalised, and a loss of control.

From a labour consideration, induction of labour can produce uterine hyper-stimulation (1–5 per cent) (NICE, 2008), uterine rupture (WHO, 2011), fetal distress (De Jong *et al.*, 1997), restricted mobility and increased pain (Buckley, 2009).

Other physical considerations of IOL are the production of progesterone in preparation for labour. This hormone softens the pelvic ligaments and allows flexibility during birth. Buckley (2009) theorises that a large baby can be accommodated by a woman's peak levels of progesterone. However, an induced labour does not benefit from natural progesterone, the pelvis remains rigid and birth complications such as shoulder dystocia are increased. This evidence needs examining if we are suggesting induction for 'big babies' as, without the proges-terone production, a big baby and an induction of labour may be a recipe for dystocia.

Top tips for induction of labour

- Encourage the woman to research induction of labour. Accepting local literature alone is a mistake. There is a wider view. Organisations such as AIMS, NCT and Birthrights are dedicated to supporting women's choices for birth.
- Know the evidence. This is not as clear cut as you would imagine.
- Statements like 'the incidence of stillbirth doubles after 42 weeks' are not helpful. Women need the figures to be able to make informed choice.
- Women and babies often do not gestate to 43 weeks. A couple of days are often all that is required.
- Encourage oxytocin production in the hospital environment (Chapter 4).
- Discuss ways of remaining mobile with intervention.
- Reinforce the woman's ability to birth.

Be aware that many women feel the need to 'encourage things along'. Their alternative induction methods may include raspberry leaf tea (NOT a form of induction), sex, curry, pineapple, acupuncture, evening primrose oil capsules and blue cohosh. Many of these have no evidence base, and some such as blue cohosh are dangerous.

Odent (2009) argues that there are no natural methods of induction. If a method is effective, it means that it is not natural, because it has preceded the signals given by the baby.

BOX 10.3 KERRY AND MIKE'S INDUCTION

My husband, Mike, and I very much enjoyed the hypnobirthing classes we attended at the hospital during February and continued to practise the techniques of massage and relaxation along with affirmations and soothing music every day. I looked forward to this time each day as it was a lovely calm time and a nice activity to do – working together, leading up to the birth.

I wrote a birth plan which included all the hypnobirthing techniques we had learnt and access to a birthing pool.

As it turned out, despite my best efforts to get things started(!) I went over my due date and was offered an induction 12 days later.

I tried questioning whether I could go on trying to get things started naturally for another couple of the days, but the doctor at the hospital advised me that I had less chance of having to have an emergency C-Section if I had the induction sooner rather than later. And he also pointed out that they would rather induce me on a Wednesday (day 12) than a Friday (day 14) as there are less staff around at the weekend! So I didn't argue with him and went ahead with the induction that day.

During that night I started to feel some pains but these came to nothing unfortunately, so we went back into the hospital on Thursday at 4pm and attempted to be induced again, this time with the gel. Unlike the day before, I immediately started to have mild surges while strapped up to the monitor.

These gentle surges continued through the afternoon. We went for a long walk around the hospital to help get things moving and then, once back on the ward, we were timing the surges. Every time I had one, Mike used a variety of the massage techniques we had learnt and practised, he also read the relaxation scripts and we were making use of a birthing ball and listening to the relaxing soundtrack I had made on my iPhone.

It wasn't ideal on the ward as we didn't have much room to use the ball and had to keep the music very low so as not to disturb the other ladies, but we knew I had to stay there as part of the induction process, so made the best of it.

We continued managing the surges in this way into the evening and, although I would have ideally preferred to have been at home, I felt calm, relaxed and happy that Mike and I were working as a team towards the birth. At 10pm, one of the staff gave me a painful examination, which showed I was still only 1–2cm dilated.

I was disappointed that I was not any further along, but mainly because I started to feel anxious that Mike would be sent home. We asked one of the staff if it would be possible for him to stay and explained that we were hypnobirthing. There were only two other ladies in the bay that night and as we were being very quiet I thought they might allow it. Unfortunately, the midwife came back a short time later and said she had checked with the matron and Mike would have to be sent home.

Neither of us was happy about this at all, but he duly left for home at about 11pm. I then got ready for bed and tried to relax. Almost immediately, the surges seemed to become much more intense and I was struggling to deal with them. By this time, the bay was in darkness and we were expected to go to sleep. I didn't want to make a fuss, but as the surges became stronger and stronger (coming about every 3 minutes) I rang my bell and asked if I could have something for the pain. I was offered a couple of paracetamol, which of course had no effect whatsoever. I tried to sleep, but it seemed that the second I would drop off, I would get another surge, which became increasingly hard for me to deal with.

During this time, I started to get increasingly anxious and frightened, as I wondered how I was going to make it through the night, putting up with this level of pain every few minutes. I guessed the staff obviously thought I had some time before things kicked off properly, as I was barely open at all at 10pm, so I had no idea how long this would go on for and, being my first, didn't know what was normal.

However, I could hear members of staff attending the ladies either side of my bed and was convinced they must have heard how loud and fast my breathing was (in order to deal with the pain) and may have guessed that I was struggling and was perhaps more along than they thought I was.

At about 2.30am I was in a pretty terrible state, feeling like my lower parts were out of control and, fearing that I was going to have an accident, managed somehow to make it to the loo. On the way back, I stopped at the nurses' station and said that I felt like I needed to push. They seemed mildly interested in this and said someone would come and examine me. Even though the previous exam was agony and I thought this was going to be the same (so wondered how I would put up with that level of pain – the exam and the surge), I welcomed it, as I desperately needed something to happen. Of course I was hoping that I would be far enough along to go down to the delivery suite but, failing that, I was even hoping for the possibility that they would somehow know the baby was getting distressed and I would have to have an emergency C-Section. Under normal circumstances, this was my worst-case scenario, but I was feeling so awful, I just wanted something (anything) to change.

I don't think I'm being overly dramatic to say I couldn't have cared if I had died at that moment!

Finally, about 2.45am someone came over to examine me. To my relief it was painless and then she announced that I was ready to go down to delivery and I could ring my husband who may or may not make it! Luckily, we only live a short walk from the hospital, so I was pretty sure he would make it, but would have been beside myself if we had lived a long way away. The nurse that examined me then went away without saying anything else and I was left to ring Mike myself (although I could barely speak!) and sat on the edge of the bed wondering when someone was going to come back for me and if I had to pick my own bags up!

About 10 minutes later, they eventually came back with a chair to wheel me down to the delivery room and luckily we met Mike in the corridor as we came out of the lift.

He said I looked like I'd had a stroke – so I must have looked a bit of a state! It turned out I was fully dilated then, so no wonder I was feeling such intense pain over those few hours, while I was alone and frightened on the ward.

Mike went back upstairs to get the rest of my stuff and then came down to the delivery room. I was met by two lovely midwives (one was a student) who were immediately onboard with the hypnobirthing – they had the music on their iPod and I instantly felt happier and relieved that I now had a team of people (two midwives and Mike) to help me birth my baby.

Everyone says you don't remember the pain of childbirth and I don't remember it in the delivery room (when it must have been more intense building up to the birth) but will **never** forget it on the ward. This shows the difference I felt psychologically, which is what the hypnobirthing is all about!

Mike then re-started the massage and relaxation scripts and I started to do the proper breathing again (which had previously gone completely out of the window!).

So, with the help of the midwives, we were able to pick up where we left off. Our baby boy, Jenson, was born just over 2 hours later.

He was 8lb 11oz. I didn't have any pain relief as it almost felt easy after my experience a few hours earlier and only had gas and air to stitch up a bad tear I had afterwards.

Although we couldn't have the waterbirth I had wanted, the room was lovely and I was able to move about in different positions, and the midwives were fantastic and were wonderful at assisting with the hypnobirthing techniques.

I have to say all the midwives we encountered were absolutely brilliant, from the two in the delivery room, to the one that assisted me immediately after the birth and those on the ward the following day. But I obviously feel differently about the night staff on that ward, from what I perceive as a lack of care through their failure to monitor me more closely, to their decision to send Mike home when, ironically, he was helping do their job for them!

I don't like having to send negative feedback, and most of the experience at the hospital was great, but I feel it is important for me to draw attention to my experience on the ward that night as it completely undermines the whole ethos of the hypnobirthing. So it feels like some parts of the hospital are teaching these wonderful techniques, while other parts are undermining it. The hypno-birthing team needs to be aware of this and I hope my feedback will help avoid this situation happening to anyone else in the future.

Continuous monitoring

Continuous cardiotocography (CTG) is a technological norm in every hospital in the UK. However the benefits of this procedure are still being argued over. As CTG monitoring is so imbedded in practice, it would be considered unethical to conduct research based on some women not being offered CTG monitoring. NICE (2014) states, 'There is therefore no high-quality evidence about the size of the benefit or harm derived from the use of cardiotocography compared with intermittent auscultation, either in individual cases or across a whole population.'

As midwives, we follow guidelines that recommend CTG for some women. We gain consent from the woman, but often do not have a full conversation with her discussing the iatrogenic risks of CTG. Women experiencing any intervention that involves continuous monitoring may find that they are physically challenged as it is often conducted on the bed. Being in the hospital environment creates the expectation of being on the bed. The advantages of being upright and mobile are well documented. Walsh (2012) suggests discussing the risks of a woman remaining in the supine position. These include decreased fetal oxygenation, lower pH, increased abnormal fetal heart patterns, longer second stage, more likelihood of having other interventions such as

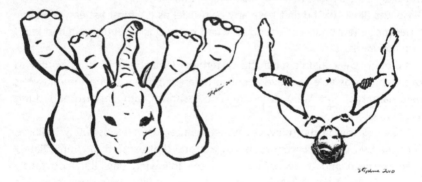

FIGURE 10.1 Unrestricted movement
Source: © Stephanie Larson, founder Dancing For Birth™, www.dancingforbirth.com. Reproduced with kind permission of Stephanie Larson, Founder Dancing For Birth™, www.dancingforbirth.com.

epidural, syntocinon, episiotomy and instrumental birth, less desire to bear down, smaller outlet diameters and more severe pain (De Jong *et al.*, 1997). Women can feel defeated by intervention and resign themselves to a less active labour. However, in my experience the midwife can also 'label' the complex birth and will often be content for the woman to be bed bound. The challenge of active birth with IV fluids, belt monitors and catheters seems too overwhelming for all but the most committed.

The physical disadvantages of bed birth are well documented, but continuous monitoring also has an impact on birth psychology. When the labouring woman knows that her body functions are continuously monitored, it leads to stimulation of her neocortex. Stimulating the neocortex risks making the labour longer, more difficult and therefore more dangerous (Odent, 2009). Mobility is associated with freedom, choice and instinct. Using telemetry wherever possible will enable monitoring for those women for whom it is essential. Understanding the guidelines and using clinical judgement will improve the woman's experience of monitoring. NICE guidance 2014 states:

- Admission monitoring for straightforward pregnancy is not required.
- Amniotomy alone is not a requirement for continuous CTG.
- Pre labour rupture of membranes requires fetal assessment at contact and at 24 hours post rupture.

Hypnobirth can be perceived as non-intervention and therefore fits the homebirth model. However, the woman who experiences birth in an obstetric unit or in a theatre will need and value the techniques the most. As we see more women access hypnobirth, the diversity of labours will be evident. Hypnobirth is for all births, and all births deserve the hypnobirth philosophy.

References

Albers, L. (1999). The duration of labour in healthy women. *Journal of Perinatology*, 19(2), 114–119.

APA (2015, October 10th). *Collins English dictionary – Complete and unabridged 10th edition.* Dictionary.com: http://dictionary.reference.com/browse/obstetric. Retrieved October 11th 2015.

BirthchoiceUK (2012). *Birthchoice UK.* www.birthchoiceuk.com/Professionals/index.html. Retrieved November 18th 2012.

Buckley, S. (2009). *Gentle birth, gentle mothering* (1st edn). New York: Celestial Arts.

Cartwright, A. (1979). *The dignity of labour? A study of childbearing and induction.* London: Tavistock Publications Ltd.

Dagustun, J. (2012). Beware the dead baby card. *AIMS Journal*, 33–37.

Davies, S. (2011). A longer labour and birth … one size does not fit all. In D. Sylvie (ed.), *Promoting normal birth. Research, reflections and guidelines* (pp. 44–51). Chester Le Street: Fresh Heart Publishing.

Davis-Floyd, R. (1992). *Birth as an American rite of passage* (1st edn). Los Angeles: University of California Press.

De Jong, P. J., Johanson, R. B. and Blaxen, P. (1997). Randomised trial comparing the upright and supine positions for the second stage of labour. *British Journal of Obstetrics and Gynaecology*, 104(5), 567–571.

Downe, S., Gyte, G. M. L., Dahlen, H.G. and Singata, M. (2013). Routine vaginal examinations for assessing progress of labour to improve outcomes for women and babies at term. London: Cochrane Database of Systematic Reviews.

Edmonds, D. L. and Byrne, D. K. (1997). Clinical method for evaluating progress in the first stage of labour. *Lancet*, 335(8681), 122.

Friedman, E. (1954). The graphic analysis of labor. *American Journal of Obstetrics and Gynecology*, 68(6), 1568–1575.

Frye, A. (2004). *Holistic Midwifery* (2nd edn, Vol. 2). Oregon: Labrys Press.

Gatward, H., Simpson, M., Woodhart, L. and Colleen-Stainton, M. (2010). Women's experiences of being induced for post-date pregnancy. *Women and Birth*, March 23rd (1), 3–9.

Green, J. (1993). Expectations and experiences of pain in labor: Findings from a large prospective study. *Birth*, 20(2), 65–72.

Hobbs, L. (1998). Assessing cervical dilatation without VEs: Watching the purple line. *The Practicing Midwife*, 34–35.

Kitzinger, S. (1978). *Some mothers' experiences of induced labour*. London: National Childbirth Trust.

Levy, V. (1999). Maintaining equilibrium: A grounded theory study of the processes involved when women make informed choices during pregnancy. *Midwifery*, 109–119.

Lewis, B., Rana, S. and Crook, E. (1975). Patient response to induction of labour. *The Lancet*, 1197.

Lothian, J. (2008). Choice, autonomy, and childbirth education. *The Journal of Perinatal Education*, 35–38.

Naaktgeboren, C. (1979). Behavioural aspects of parturition. *Animal Reproductive Science*, 155–166.

NICE (2014). *Intrapartum care: Care of healthy women and their babies during childbirth*. London: National Institute for Health and Care Excellence.

NICE (2008). *Induction of labour*. London: National Institute for Clinical Excellence.

Odent, M. (2009, September 4th). The midwives of Bethany Womens Healthcare. Birth Physiology: http://azmidwives.blogspot.co.uk. Retrieved March 19th 2013.

Schmid, V. (2011). *Promoting normal birth. Research, reflections and guidelines*. Chester Le Street: Fresh Heart Publishing.

Shepherd, A., Cheyne, H., Kennedy, S., McIntosh, C., Styles, M. and Niven, C. (2010). The purple line as a measure of labour progress: A longitudinal study. *BMC Pregnancy and Childbirth*.

Uvnas-Moberg, K., Arn, I. and Magnusson, D. (2005). The psychobiology of emotion: The role of oxytocinergic system. *International Journal of Behavioral Medicine*, 59–65.

Walsh, D. (2012). *Evidence and skills for normal labour and birth* (2nd edn). London: Routledge.

Wertz, D. and Wertz, R. (1989). *Lying in: A history of childbirth in America* (expanded edn). New Haven, Connecticut: Yale University Press.

Westfall, R. E. and Benoit, C. (2004). The rhetoric of 'natural' in natural childbirth: Childbearing women's perspectives on prolonged pregnancy and induction of labour. *Social Science and Medicine*, 1397–1408.

Wickham, S. (2010). Reflecting on risk assessment. *MIDIRS*, 50–51.

World Health Organization (WHO) (2011). *Induction of labour*. Geneva: WHO Press.

Zhang, J., Troendle, J. F. and Yancey, M. K. (2002). Reassessing the labor curve in nulliparous women. *American Journal of Obstetrics and Gynecology*, 824–828.

11

IS A PAIN-FREE BIRTH POSSIBLE?

If you spend enough years supporting women in labour, there will be those who stick in your mind: the woman who arrived looking as if she were not labouring at all and gave birth 10 minutes later. The ones who make it look 'easy'. These may have been hypnobirthers. They may not have been. For some women, childbirth is pain free. The question that is always central in my mind is, if one woman can do it, why can't all women?

Much of the appeal of hypnobirth early on was its promise of the possibility of pain-free birth. As this concept is so far removed from what most women's expectations of birth are, it is almost impossible to resist exploring. These days most hypnobirth courses will talk in realistic terms of a more comfortable birth experience. We do not promise women in our classes a pain-free experience. Nor do we rule it out.

There is no doubt that many women have experienced pain during birth. This is especially true for off-plan births, when the straightforward birth becomes something else. However, this discussion around pain and birth concentrates on normal physiology.

Childbirth is often not discussed without using the pain word. There are no common alternative superlatives to replace the description of pain. Pain as a description for birth is imbedded in cultural normality. When meeting a new hypnobirth group for the first time, pain, and the expectation of it, is a major talking point. It is interesting that one small word can be used to describe such a range of experiences. Period pain, migraine pain, back pain, tooth pain, post-operative pain, emotional pain and labour pain. Each event will be experienced completely differently, and yet our language offers no variation. Most pain is seen as pathological. However, for many women birth is a normal physiological event. As we know the effect of language and expectation on the mind, to continue to characterise labour as painful is limiting. During the last 5 years I have taught hundreds of couples hypnobirth. Most share their birth stories and the range and diversity of experiences is vast. For many women, they would accept that there was pain, but found it completely manageable. One woman described it as 'a bit gripey'. Many did not realise it was labour until almost the end of first stage. For a small group of women, there was no pain attached to birth. Birth was not without sensation, but they would not have described it as painful.

Interestingly, there is reluctance in society to accept this type of experience. I remember a midwife who happens to be very petite and gave birth to a beautiful five-and-a-half pound baby using hypnobirth. This was a perfect size baby for her body. However, when she told other midwives that birth had been comfortable, they all remarked that it was a small baby that made it so easy! There seems a real reluctance to accept anything other than the badge-of-honour, dramatic, screaming version of birth. Women who experience anything else are a fluke, lucky or delusional. Women who attend hypnobirth classes often plan an analgesia-free birth. They report feeling reluctant to share this with friends and family for fear of being smirked at and judged, and the attitude of 'why be a hero?' The relationship with birth and pain is a complex one, and everyone has an opinion.

Danielle says:

> From the moment I found out I was pregnant I panicked and worried constantly that something bad would happen and I was terrified of giving birth. It was recommended by my midwife that I took a hypnobirthing class. I just want to recommend this class to anyone who is anxious about their pregnancy or labour. It was fantastic and made me so chilled out about everything. I stopped panicking and felt so calm. It also got my husband really involved, which was lovely as we had to practise relaxation techniques at home. I kept saying to people that, although I still didn't know how I would cope with labour on the day, at least I felt relaxed leading up to it and that was worth it for me.

Attitudes towards pain

The woman

When teaching a hypnobirth group, there is an opportunity to open up discussion around pain. As a hypnobirth teacher I do not want to focus on the pain aspect or suggest that is what they are going to experience. However, I do feel there is value in a discussion around their beliefs, as it can enable us to move on. Many of the hypnobirth brands do not offer such an opportunity, but as a midwife I see it as a starting point towards a comfortable birth. Denying that pain exists in childbirth lessens the credibility of hypnobirth. The couples all know someone who had a genuinely painful experience. It may be their second or third child and, if they experienced previous pain in labour themselves, then discussing 'pain-free' birth is a stretch. The question is, Why do women experience pain in labour? Their answers:

- It's like birthing a watermelon.
- Big object, small hole.
- Because it's supposed to hurt.
- Fear.
- Because god is a man.
- Tearing, ripping.
- Because I believe it will hurt.
- Because we walk on two legs and not four.
- Small pelvis.
- Low pain threshold.

There are many variations on the theme, but parents come with their own ideas about pain and birth. It is good practice to acknowledge that for some women birth is painful, especially off-plan birth. It is also equally important to acknowledge that women do give birth comfortably.

BOX 11.1 JODI AND JAMES'S STORY

Before attending your hypnobirthing class I was determined to have a C-section and as many drugs as available. I can't believe I had a natural birth and I enjoyed every moment.

Here's my hypnobirthing story …

When I fell pregnant, my midwife visited and asked what type of birth I wanted. I responded with 'drugs' and a 'C-section'. When she asked why, I explained I was terrified of birth and I had a low pain threshold. I felt a mixed bag of emotions. I felt guilty that I was scared of bringing my child in to the world. I felt scared (after all, so many people had shared their horror story with me).

I also felt powerless, as no one knew how the birth would go. My midwife suggested hypnobirthing lessons and I agreed … soon I realised that labour and birth didn't need to be a horrible, daunting and painful experience.

On Tuesday evening I felt some surges. I breathed through them and because they weren't painful I assumed it was Braxton Hicks. I stayed downstairs watching movies, timing the surges during the night. At first they were every 17 minutes, then reducing down to 10 minutes, 8 minutes …. And by 4am I realised the surges were every 3 minutes. I made some toast with raspberry jam on and coffee and I took it up to my husband who was asleep at 4am and I told him that 'I think I'm in labour …. But it doesn't hurt!?!'

I had a shower, whilst he ate his toast, and I stayed very calm, breathing through the surges.

On the way to the hospital I called the ward, who said that I should have called before I left home as I probably wouldn't have needed to come in. They said that, as I was nearly at the hospital, I should go in but warned I would probably be sent home.

As I walked in to the hospital I reminded myself how the smell of the hospital resembled 'Life' and 'healing'. When I arrived on the birthing unit I was asked to take a seat. After 10 minutes I went into a birthing suite. I was chatting to the midwife and used the birthing ball to ease my surges. In fact the birthing ball eased them completely. The midwife told me it was highly unlikely that I was in labour as I wouldn't have been able to have a conversation if I was and I would be (as she demonstrated) bent over the bed unable to speak. I was a bit disappointed and braced myself to go home. The midwife did an examination and to our astonishment she found I was 2cm dilated. I stayed in the birthing room feeling very relaxed and within 45 minutes I wanted to push. My husband called the midwife who examined me again. I was now 10cm dilated but I was not feeling any pain. I was offered gas and air which I took (mainly because I was a little nervous).

I stayed in stage 2 of my birth for 22 minutes. There was not time to fill the birthing pool and instead I gave birth on all fours. It's incredibly embarrassing to say but a big worry for me was that I pooped during the birth and that is exactly what I thought I had done … I was devastated and said to the midwife how sorry I was. The midwife assured me that I hadn't and instead it was the head which I had delivered. I couldn't believe it! It was unbelievable that it was nearly over. All those months of worry and it was a pain-free and wonderful birth. I wish I had enjoyed my pregnancy more and stopped stressing over the birth.

Hypnobirthing was incredible and a massive contributing factor to how I was home within 10 hours of arriving at the hospital. I cannot thank you enough or explain how much this has been life changing.

Pain could be seen as transformational. Anthropologist Margaret Mead observed that birth can be seen as both painful and dangerous or an interesting, enriching experience, depending on the culture (Mead, 2001 and Schmid, 2011). The attitude and expectation of the woman anticipating birth can in part determine the experience. There are psychological processes that may underpin an approach to pain. It may be explained using self-efficacy theory (Bandura, 1977). Self-efficacy refers to a person's judgement of their capability to carry out certain behaviours. The greater the perceived self-efficacy, then the more likely it is that an individual will actually behave in that way. Evidence from laboratory-induced pain and clinical pain studies suggests that a person's coping self-efficacy can mediate the effectiveness of different psychological coping strategies. In a study of pain tolerance to the cold pressor test, Bandura found that training in cognitive coping strategies significantly increased perceived self-efficacy, both to withstand and reduce pain compared with a placebo or control. Similarly, it can be argued that hypnobirth today allows women to access cognitive coping strategies. Schmid (2011) discusses the need for pain in transitional experiences. There are some cultures where male societies have created initiation rites to mark the arrival of puberty, fatherhood, war or marriage. These often involve men subjecting themselves to physical or psychological pain, emerging on the other side stronger, wiser, transformed. The addition of pain confirms the belief that comfortable and easy are somehow less valuable – 'no pain, no gain' is a common maxim.

Linear to this is the popular belief that mothers who birth through painful labours are somehow transformed into confident, strong, empowered mothers. Leap *et al.* (2010) say:

'The pain of labour marks the enormous change that is occurring in a woman's life – her transition to motherhood; her joy at becoming a mother can be heightened by the contrast with the pain of labour.'

Donegan (2006) argues for the mothers who birth without discomfort: Are they less empowered, less confident mothers? Does an easy experience result in less value?

The care provider

Can the midwife/care provider influence the woman's perception of pain in labour? Anecdotally, the answer is yes. The care provider's own experience of birth, her attitude to analgesia and belief in normality all have an impact on the experience. An understanding of hypnobirth can facilitate the quiet, undisturbed, relaxed labour that the couple are looking for. Many midwives would argue that they are impartial, non-biased supporters of birth. I would argue that, as individuals, with our own experiences and preferences, we cannot be impartial. We can, however, be aware of our own bias, reflective and open minded to alternative experiences. Maybe it is time to embrace our subjectivity, be honest about our bias and enable the mother–midwife relationship to flourish into 'a good fit'. Women and their birth partners often know long before the midwife if they are not on the same page. Often there can be a resolution, but sometimes the only answer is to offer a different care provider.

An overview of pain in labour by Leap *et al.* (2010) highlights attitudes to pain in labour and suggests that they could be separated into two paradigms, that of 'working with pain' and that of 'pain relief'. This can be a good starting point for pain discussion, as most women and midwives will have a leaning towards one paradigm or the other. The midwife's attitude, her language and even her body language can support or defeat a labour.

Four quotes from midwives caring for women using hypnosis in labour:

'It will probably be the worst pain you have ever felt, but it's worth it.'
'Oh you're one of those hypnobirthers, are you?'
'Why are you putting yourself through this? Let me get you an epidural.'
'I will examine you in an hour or so; it's very likely you are still only 4cm' (10 minutes before baby was breathed out in a busy post-/antenatal ward).

By contrast, Becky says:

Clare was very supportive of our hypnobirthing plan and did not try to intervene or interrupt during the times that she could see I was concentrating.

We barely knew she was there. The lights were dimmed and it was a very tranquil environment, just as I had imagined it to be.

Alex says:

> Cheryl explained that she was actually a 'high-risk' midwife and rarely worked in the midwifery unit so didn't come across hypnobirthing that often. With regular checks from Melissa (the student), she was happy to leave me to it as per my birth plan unless I told her otherwise. A connection is important and I felt immediately comfortable with both of them, especially as they seemed to respect and support my plan.

Joy says:

> One of the midwives had witnessed a hypnobirth before and had also seen the film *Microbirth* so was totally convinced about the enormous benefits of having as natural a birth as possible. This was a huge relief. The other midwife reassured me she would make sure things were as quiet as possible and wouldn't use the words 'pain' or 'contraction'.

Worryingly, many couples arrive at antenatal classes wanting information on 'pain relief'. More worryingly, traditional 'parentcraft' classes will focus on analgesia available and interventions that the woman may experience. To perpetuate the myth that there is pain relief available reinforces the woman's belief that if she cannot cope the medical profession can solve it. There is very little we can offer a woman in labour that is safe and risk free and will remove all pain. Normal birth is not supposed to be 'solved', and the sensations she experiences are what she is physiologically capable of. What women need are internal resources, confidence in their ability and coping strategies that enable them to move through the journey.

Pain and the experience of it in childbirth is a complex topic. A woman's sensation can be influenced by many things:

- past experiences of pain
- cultural conditioning
- expectations
- media and social influence
- antenatal preparation
- fear/tension
- support in labour
- self-efficacy
- knowledge.

Much of the criticism levelled at the hypnobirth world includes the denial of the existence of pain in labour. Having looked at how expectation, language and beliefs affect pain, you will understand why the focus is on comfortable birth as opposed to painful birth. For some, the popular mythology of hypnobirth is of a woman home birthing, sitting in a yoga pose with a smile on her face as her baby easily slips out. This may be a reality for some women. However, for many women, birth takes place out of the home environment. The hypnobirth woman understands that all choices of analgesia are still available to her. She also understands that birth will take all her focus and concentration. Labour sensation is both appropriate and relevant. We do not claim to anticipate how she will experience those sensations. What we do know is that pain is limiting terminology and, when we offer up alternatives, the hypnobirth woman embraces the experience.

References

Bandura, A. (1977). Self efficacy: Towards a unifying theory of behavioural change. *Psychological Review*, 191–215.

Donegan, T. (2006). Hypnobirthing: Instinctive birthing through relaxation. *Midwifery Today*.

Leap, N., Sandall, J., Buckland, S. and Huber, U. (2010). Journey to confidence: Women's experiences of pain in labour and relational continuity of care. *Journal of Midwifery and Women's Health*, 55(3) May–Jun, 234–242.

Mead, M. (2001). *Male and female*. New York: Harper Perennial.

Schmid, V. (2011). *Birth pain*. Chester Le Street: Fresh Heart Publishing.

INDEX

Page numbers in *italics* refer to figures. Page numbers in **bold** refer to tables.

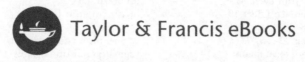